The Institute of Biology's
Studies in Biology no. 60

The Secretion of Milk

Ben Mepham
B.Sc., Ph.D.
Lecturer in Animal Physiology,
University of Nottingham

Edward Arnold

Printed in Great Britain by
The Camelot Press Ltd, Southampton

General Preface to the Series

It is no longer possible for one textbook to cover the whole field of Biology and to remain sufficiently up to date. At the same time teachers and students at school, college or university need to keep abreast of recent trends and know where the significant developments are taking place.

To meet the need for this progressive approach the Institute of Biology has for some years sponsored this series of booklets dealing with subjects specially selected by a panel of editors. The enthusiastic acceptance of the series by teachers and students at school, college and university shows the usefulness of the books in providing a clear and up-to-date coverage of topics, particularly in areas of research and changing views.

Among features of the series are the attention given to methods, the inclusion of a selected list of books for further reading and, wherever possible, suggestions for practical work.

Reader's comments will be welcomed by the author or the Education Office of the Institute.

1975   The Institute of Biology
41 Queen's Gate
London, SW7 5HU

Preface

The subject of this book receives scant attention in most introductory texts on mammalian biology, usually being relegated to the last paragraph of the last chapter, that on reproduction. I have attempted to remedy this situation and to show that not only is lactation a process of great importance in mammalian species, but also that recent discoveries made by scientists studying milk secretion are of significance to our understanding of the fundamental mechanisms controlling biosynthetic and secretory processes.

I am indebted to Dr. J. L. Linzell for reading the draft manuscript and for constructive criticism.

Sutton Bonington, 1975   T. B. M.

Contents

1 Evolution of the Mammary Gland and its Secretion

1.1 Introduction

There are reputed to be 4237 species of mammal in existence. The essential characteristic distinguishing them from other animals is the possession by the female of mammary glands, which, by secreting milk, provide a source of nutrient to the new-born. Other features usually associated with mammals, such as viviparity and the possession of a hair coat, are not shown by all species of the class. Milk secretion, however, has a significance which extends beyond its purely nutritive role. Lactation constitutes one aspect of the phase of mammalian life in which maternal care of the young is necessarily at its most pronounced, and when infant-maternal behavioural interactions are likely to be of the greatest significance to the future social development of the new-born. Also, in many species, the milk secreted in the immediately *post-partum* period (termed 'colostrum') contains antibodies, which confer on the offspring an immunity to infections.

1.2 Comparative aspects of lactation

The first forms of mammalian life are believed to have emerged about 150 million years ago. It is probable that the mammary glands appeared at a time when increasing parental care of a few young was evolved as a means of ensuring species survival, as an alternative to that seen in lower animals, in which most of the large numbers of young produced perish.

The class Mammalia has three sub-classes, viz. (i) the Prototheria, containing the single order Monotremata, (ii) the Metatheria, also containing a single order, the Marsupialia, and (iii) the Eutheria (placental mammals) which constitutes over 95% of all mammals and comprises seventeen different orders. The characteristics of these sub-classes are discussed below.

1.2.1 Basic structure of the mammary gland

The mammary glands of all mammalian species have the same basic structure, which is both simple and relatively homogeneous. Milk is synthesized in specialized epithelial cells ('secretory cells') from substances absorbed from the blood. The secretory cells are grouped together in spherical sacs or 'alveoli', the milk being secreted into their lumina and then drained via a system of arborizing ducts towards the body surface. The arrangement of the alveoli and ducts, which is described as 'racemose', is reminiscent of a bunch of grapes on a twig. Groups of alveoli which are drained by a common large duct constitute a lobule, neighbouring lobules being separated by connective tissue. Collectively the secretory elements of the parenchyma are termed the 'lobulo-alveolar system' to distinguish them from the duct system, although the cells of the finer-calibre ducts are also probably capable of secretion. The glands are invariably situated beneath the skin and external to the body cavity.

A curiously analogous mode of nutrient production is shown by pigeons, in which, at the time of hatching, glands lining the crop of both the male and female parents hypertrophy and secrete 'pigeon milk'. There appears, however, to be little chemical resemblance between pigeon milk and true mammalian milk.

1.2.2 Monotremes

The duck-billed platypus is perhaps the best known species of monotreme. This animal lays eggs, and, after hatching, the young receive milk from 200 or so glands which are grouped in two areas, one on each side of the mid-line, on the ventral surface of the dam. The importance of lactation is illustrated by the fact that the young remain within the nest for 3–4 months after hatching, and with milk as the sole source of food, grow from less than 2 cm in length to about 45 cm (¾ adult size). In another species, the echidna, a pouch develops on the abdomen of the dam at the beginning of the breeding season. The eggs are transferred to the pouch and, after hatching, the young receive milk from glands, the ducts of which open into the pouch. Monotreme glands do not possess teats, the structures which in higher mammals facilitate the efficient transfer of milk from dam to offspring.

1.2.3 Marsupials

The name of this order derives from the presence of a pouch on the ventral surface of the abdomen of the female (Greek, marsupion = small purse), although it is in the relationship between the genital and urinary ducts that marsupials are most clearly distinguishable from other mammals. Marsupials are viviparous, but gestation is extremely short, usually only 3–4 weeks, and lactation plays a correspondingly more prominent role in the growth and development of the young than is the case in eutherians. An illustration of the importance of lactation in marsupials is provided by the bandicoot, which weighs only 50 mg at birth but attains a weight of 50 g within 50 days. 'The marsupial at birth is a marvellous composite of embryonic structures and precociously developed functional organs, the latter enabling it to reach the pouch, respire and gain nourishment from the mammary gland' (TYNDALE-BISCOE, 1973). The glands are usually situated within the pouch and the ducts of neighbouring lobes join and lead to the body surface via a teat. The number of separate glands varies greatly between species, ranging from two to twenty-five. Because of the relative brevity of gestation and length of lactation, kangaroos may nurse two generations of young simultaneously, the suckled glands showing quite different degrees of development and secreting milk of widely differing composition. Teats are invariably present in lactating marsupials and the young have modified buccal cavities which allow them to breathe concurrently with suckling. Indeed, the young become so firmly attached to the teats that they can only be removed with extreme difficulty.

1.2.4   Eutherians

The foetal eutherian receives nutrients *in utero* via the placenta, and at birth is relatively much more mature than is the young marsupial. Individuals of some species (e.g. the guinea-pig) can indeed survive without milk. Nevertheless, for most species milk constitutes an extremely important source of food in the immediately *post-partum* period.

In all eutherians the fully functional gland is a compound tubulo-alveolar structure demarcated into lobes and lobules by connective tissue septa. Milk produced by the secretory cells drains via the duct system into large ducts which open on to the body surface via teats or nipples: in many species the ducts open into sinuses or cisterns within the gland, which increase the capacity to store milk. The number and distribution of glands varies widely between species, e.g. in man, two on the ventral thorax; in cows, four in the inguinal region; in sows, 10–14 in pairs along the whole length of the ventral thorax and abdomen: in the coypu the glands are situated dorsally. Most of the research on the physiology and biochemistry of mammary function has been carried out on eutherian species, so that in the following text it should be assumed, unless otherwise stated, that the discussion pertains, strictly, only to such species. It is, however, important to realize that very few species have been subjected to detailed study. Most investigations have been performed either on small laboratory animals, such as the rat and mouse, or on dairy species, and these may not be at all representative of eutherians as a zoological group.

1.3   Evolution of the mammary gland

The question of the homology of the mammary gland (i.e. from which structures in non-mammalian species has the gland developed?) has intrigued biologists since the time of Darwin. Although it is conceivable that the gland was formed *de novo* at the expense of ectoderm and the underlying mesenchymal tissues, and is thus homologous to no particular non-mammalian structure, it has seemed more probable that it evolved from one or more of the skin glands which are distributed so widely over the body surface of mammals. There are three types of skin gland in mammals, each exhibiting a distinct mode of secretion of their products. In holocrine glands there is a complete degeneration of the mature cell so that the nuclear and cytoplasmic components are secreted *in toto*. This type of secretion is typical of sebaceous glands, whose product, sebum, is chiefly lipid. Eccrine glands by contrast produce an aqueous salt solution, the secretion of which does not apparently involve any loss of cellular integrity. This mode of secretion is confined to sweat glands, which by virtue of the high latent heat of vaporization of water, are an important element in thermoregulation. The third type of secretion, aprocrine secretion, is intermediate between these two extremes in that some loss of apical cytoplasm only occurs along with the secretory product. This mode of secretion is exemplified by a second type of sweat gland producing an opalescent fluid, components of which are believed, in certain species, to act as pheromones and as such are important in sexual attraction.

Controversy still exists as to whether sweat glands of this latter type or sebaceous glands are the more likely precursors of mammary glands. Apocrine sweat glands are relatively large structures with a branching duct system and possessing prominent myoepithelial cells, the contraction of which aids the expulsion of sweat from the ducts. In both these respects they are similar to mammary glands. Moreover, the apocrine mode of secretion has been observed, albeit to a slight extent only, in the mammary gland. Perhaps more pertinent is the fact that holocrine secretion does not appear to occur in the mammary gland and would in any event necessitate an almost inconceivable rate of mitosis to replenish cells degraded in secretion. On the other hand sebaceous glands are particularly prevalent in the region of hairs, their excretory ducts frequently opening into the hair follicles, a situation very similar to the relationship between mammary ducts and hair follicles in monotremes. It is not possible here to discuss all the merits of the opposing theories, but it is clear that the most widely held view is that mammary glands have evolved from apocrine sweat glands, or alternatively that both structures have evolved from a common precursor.

On this basis an attractive, though highly speculative, theory has been proposed for the origin of the mammary glands. According to this scheme the mammary areas of monotremes may be traced back to the brooding spots of reptilian ancestors. With the development of the hairy coat the rich blood supply to these areas would have favoured the rapid growth of associated skin glands. It is not unreasonable to suppose that the newly-hatched young would have licked or sucked these areas, the processes of natural selection resulting in compositional changes in the secretion, so that what we now refer to as 'milk' was evolved.

1.4   General characteristics of milk

Since milk is almost invariably the sole source of nutrient for the new-born, at least in the immediately *post-partum* period, it might be supposed that it would contain all the food materials necessary for growth and development of the young. This, however, is not always the case, even when the dam is apparently perfectly nourished. All milks, for example, show low concentrations of iron. Since this element is necessary for the formation of the respiratory pigment, haemoglobin, its inadequacy may lead to acute anaemia, as occurs in an unfortunately high proportion of neonatal piglets reared under artificial conditions, i.e. when they are unable to root in the soil. Certain species are able to offset this deficiency by drawing on iron reserves laid down in the liver during foetal development. Despite inadequacies of this nature, it is clear that milk does constitute an almost complete food for the young. It is also probably the most complete single food, a view which has been appreciated for thousands of years, and accounts in large measure for man's domestication of docile, herbivorous mammals like the cow, goat, camel and reindeer. Even now certain West African nomadic tribes are reputed to live for months exclusively on milk.

There is an enormous variation in the status of the new-born between different species of mammal. The source of this variation lies in factors such as the size and physiological maturity of the young at birth, the diet and behavioural characteristics of the dam and environmental factors, and as a consequence the requirements of the young for nutrients also differ considerably between species. Not surprisingly these varying requirements are reflected in variations in the composition and quantity of milk secreted by the dams of different species. With very few exceptions, however, milk from all species has the same basic qualitative composition. At the time of its secretion milk consists of two liquid phases, fat and water, between which are partitioned a large number of chemical compounds. In the aqueous phase, lactose (milk sugar), minerals such as calcium, phosphorus and magnesium, and water-soluble vitamins are present in simple solution, while proteins are present in colloidal suspension. The lipid phase contains fat-soluble vitamins and substances such as sterols and carotenoids. For obvious reasons most analyses of milk composition have been carried out on bovine milk, and the inevitable dependence on data from this source should be appreciated in the following sections in which the characteristics of individual milk components are discussed.

1.5   Lactose

Lactose is a disaccharide in which galactose is joined in a β linkage to the 4-position of glucose (Fig. 1–1). Although there are a few instances of the occurrence of lactose in plants, its formation in the mammary gland is apparently unique in animals.

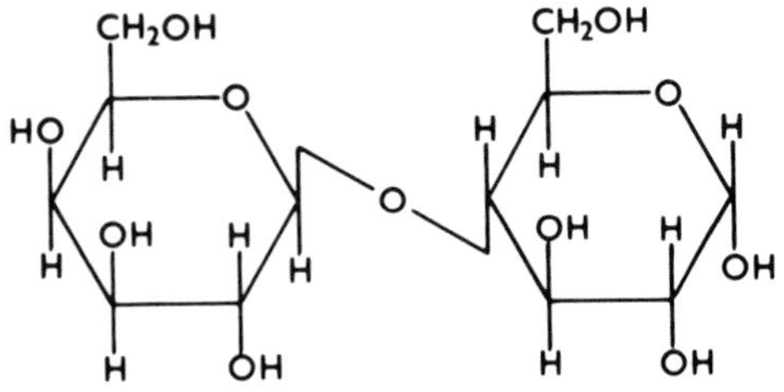

Fig. 1–1   The lactose molecule.

Lactose is split into its constituent monosaccharides under the influence of the intestinal enzyme, lactase, and since galactose can be converted to glucose, lactose may be regarded simply as a source of glucose, the oxidation of which provides energy in the form of ATP (see Chapter 3). If this is the case, glucose itself would seem to be a more suitable component of milk. It is, however, likely that certain properties of lactose have proved advantageous in the evolutionary development of mammals. In all the species which have been studied milk is isotonic with blood plasma. In terms of the energy expended in secreting milk this imposes less demand on the dam than would be the case if it were hypo- or hypertonic. Of the three major components of milk, fat, protein and lactose, only the latter, because of its low molecular weight, exerts a significant osmotic pressure. Given this situation, lactose provides nearly twice the calorific value per molecule (and hence per unit of osmotic pressure) than would glucose. Other attributes of lactose are that it provides a beneficial medium for intestinal activity regulating (i) the bacterial flora, (ii) the pH of the alimentary tract and (iii) the absorption of minerals.

In monotremes and marsupials the predominant sugars present are trisaccharides and not lactose.

1.6   Caseins

Milk proteins may be broadly classified as caseins and whey proteins. Caseins are phosphoproteins, occurring uniquely in milk, which precipitate at acid pH (pH 4.6 for bovine milk) or under the influence of the enzyme, rennin (also called chymosin), which is secreted by cells of the gastric mucosa in young ruminants. The formation of the protein clot or 'curd' in the stomach of the new-born facilitates the efficient digestion of the protein by proteolytic enzymes. In view of their high content of essential amino acids (i.e. those which cannot be synthesized in the body) caseins are an important source of substrates for protein synthesis in the new-born, but they appear also to serve another important role, i.e. in mineral transport. Casein molecules associate together in combination with Ca^{2+}, $PO_4{}^{3-}$ and Mg^{2+} ions in structures known as micelles. As a result of this, and the fact that phosphorus is attached by ester linkages to certain amino acid residues in the protein, the quantities of Ca^{2+} and $PO_4{}^{3-}$ which may be carried in milk greatly exceed the amounts present in simple aqueous solution. The significance of this is apparent when one considers that bone is very largely composed of $Ca_3(PO_4)_2$.

Using electrophoresis and other techniques it has been shown that there are several different types of casein molecule (Fig. 1–2) and that

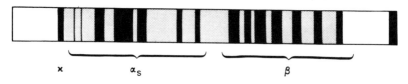

Fig. 1–2 Separation of caseins of guinea-pig milk by electrophoresis on polyacrylamide gels. Protein bands made visible by staining. Designation of casein fractions is tentative only. (Reproduced by courtesy of DR. S. R. DAVIS.)

their relative concentration in the milk of different species varies considerably. In bovine milk, caseins are classified into α_S, β and κ caseins, each group being heterogeneous. The mean molecular weights range from 20 000 to 27 000 daltons. It is believed that κ casein, which is a glycoprotein, normally stabilizes α_S casein against precipitation by Ca^{2+} ions. κ casein is, however, split by the action of rennin, so that in the stomach the micellar structure breaks down and clotting occurs.

1.7 Whey proteins

In contrast to the caseins, whey proteins are not precipitated at acid pH. These proteins are of two types, viz. those which like the caseins are specific to milk, and serum proteins, which are present in both blood and milk.

In the former category is the major whey protein of bovine milk, β lactoglobulin (a misnomer, because it is, in fact, an albumin). The protein has a number of genetic variants, so that bovine milk may contain one or a mixture of two or three of these. The protein has so far only been detected in the milks of artiodactyl (cloven-hooved) species. No function other than that of providing amino acids on digestion has been ascribed to it.

α lactalbumin is also a specific milk protein, but it appears to be present in the milks of virtually all species. Like the other proteins it is a source of amino acids to the new-born, and is rich in the essential amino acid tryptophan. In 1966 a discovery was made concerning the intracellular function of α lactalbumin, which not only indicated that it had a significance considerably greater than the purely nutritive, but also demonstrated that it performed a role hitherto not described in animal tissues. The terminal step in the sequence of reactions involved in lactose biosynthesis is catalysed by the enzyme 'lactose synthetase'. BRODBECK and EBNER, in the U.S.A., showed that this enzyme consists of two dissociable proteins, designated A and B, and that B protein is identical with α lactalbumin. The A protein alone catalyses a quite different reaction, but in the presence of α lactalbumin (the 'specifier protein') its substrate specificity is altered and lactose produced. Modifications of enzyme activity of this type have previously only been observed in bacteria. The implications of this unique property of α lactalbumin will be discussed in later chapters.

Serum albumin is also present in milk at very low concentrations (approx. 1% of total bovine milk proteins). The protein is identical with blood serum albumin and would thus appear to be transferred directly from blood to milk.

Proteins of the globulin fraction of whey are of importance in some species as carriers of immune antibodies. Immunity, or more precisely, 'resistance' to infectious diseases, may be either active or passive. Active resistance implies that the tissues of an organism respond to the presence of a foreign protein ('antigen') by manufacturing antibodies, i.e. proteins which, by causing agglutination or lysis of the foreign material, neutralize its toxic effects. Young mammals depend for resistance on immunity which is transferred passively from the dam. Antibodies are carried on certain proteins of the γ globulin fraction of blood plasma which are known as immunoglobulins. In some species (e.g. man, rabbit and guinea-pig) immunoglobulins are transferred across the placenta, so that immunity is acquired *in utero*. However, because of a difference in the structure of the placental membranes this route is not operative in many domesticated species (e.g. cow, sheep, goat, horse and pig), and it is in these species that the immunoglobulin content of milk is vitally important. Immunoglobulins are present in colostrum at much higher concentration than later in lactation. Moreover in the first few days *post-partum* the gut of the young mammal is permeable to proteins, so that antibodies are absorbed into the blood unchanged. Techniques of protein separation, such as electrophoresis, have allowed identification of different immunoglobulin (Ig) fractions. Fractions IgG and IgM are present in the colostrum of cows, pigs and sheep, while in humans and rabbits IgA is the main component.

1.8 Milk fat

The fat of milk is present in the form of globules (mean diameter 3 μm in bovine milk), which are largely composed of triglycerides. Each globule is surrounded by a hydrophilic surface layer, the fat-globule membrane, which is composed of a complex mixture of compounds such as phospholipids, carotenoids, vitamin A and cholesterol, and which serves to maintain the fat in an emulsified state. Triglycerides are derivatives of glycerol in which a fatty acid forms an ester link with each of the three hydroxyl groups (Fig. 1–3). The fatty acids present are either saturated or unsaturated, the latter possessing one or more C=C bonds and thus being capable of combining with one or more pairs of H atoms.

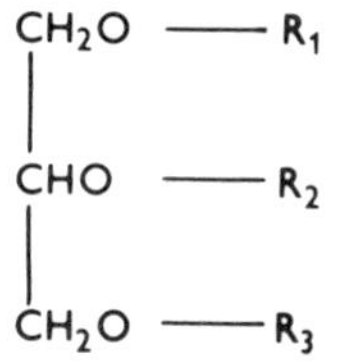

$$
\begin{array}{l}
CH_2O \longrightarrow R_1 \\
| \\
CHO \longrightarrow R_2 \\
| \\
CH_2O \longrightarrow R_3
\end{array}
$$

Fig. 1–3   Triglyceride structure. R_1, R_2 and R_3 are fatty acids.

Most saturated fatty acids of milk fat contain an even number of carbon atoms. These range from the C_4 acid (butyric) to the C_{20} (arachidic), the general formula being $CH_3(CH_2)_n.COOH$, where n is an even number ranging from 2 to 18. In addition bovine milk contains approximately 2% of saturated fatty acids with an odd number of carbon atoms and a similar proportion of methyl-branched chain saturated fatty acids with odd and even numbers of carbon atoms. Of the unsaturated fatty acids, oleic acid (mono-unsaturated C_{18}) is by far the most prevalent, but linoleic (di-unsaturated) and linolenic (tri-unsaturated) acids also occur in milk. The presence of the latter two may be particularly important, since like many of the amino acids, the body is unable to synthesize them and they are consequently essential dietary constituents.

There are certain clearly-defined species differences in milk fat composition. Ruminant milks characteristically have a high proportion of short chain, i.e. less than C_{10}, fatty acids, while those of most non-ruminants have virtually no short-chain acids. Palmitic (C_{16} saturated) and oleic (C_{18} mono-unsaturated) acids appear to be present in most milks, but in some, e.g. rabbit milk, caprylic (C_8 saturated) and capric (C_{10} saturated) acids predominate.

1.9   Composition of the milks of different species

We have seen that, apart from a basic qualitative similarity, there are wide variations between the compositions of milks of different species. Table 1 summarizes data on the major milk components of several species.

Table 1   Compositions of the milks of different species. The data are average figures expressed in g/100 cm³ or g/100 g milk. (* In these species the figures quoted are for 'milk sugar', which is chiefly trisaccharide.) (From JENNES, R. and SLOAN, R. E. (1970) Dairy Sci. Abstr. 32.)

Species	Total Solids	Fat	Casein	Whey protein	Lactose
Monotremata					
Echidna	—	9.6	7.3	5.2	0.9*
Marsupialia					
Quokka	13.4	0.9	2.2	1.8	3.4*
Eutheria					
Domestic rabbit	32.8	18.3		13.9	2.1
House mouse	29.3	13.1	7.0	2.0	3.0
Norway rat	21.0	10.3	6.4	2.0	2.6
Human	12.4	3.8	0.4	0.6	7.0
Cow	12.7	3.7	2.8	0.6	4.8
Goat	13.2	4.5	2.5	0.4	4.1
Sheep	19.3	7.4	4.6	0.9	4.8
Horse	11.2	1.9	1.3	1.2	6.2
Blue whale	57.1	42.3	7.2	3.7	1.3
Grey seal	67.7	53.2		11.2	2.6
Polar bear	47.6	33.1	7.1	3.8	0.3

It might be imagined that such variations have evolved solely to meet the differing nutritional requirements of the young of different species, a view which finds expression in the common assertion that 'mother's milk must be best'. In reality the situation is probably much more complex, involving factors such as the metabolic strain imposed by lactation on the dam, and the diet, behavioural and environmental characteristics of the species. The question of the suitability of the milk for the young thus resolves itself into a 'chicken and egg' problem.

Nevertheless, milk composition must be determined in some way, and since the nineteenth century attempts have been made to explain inter-species variations in terms of a few simple generalizations. Many of the earlier conclusions have, in the light of more recent data, proved untenable. It is also questionable whether comparison of milks on the basis of the concentrations of constituents is always appropriate, since the total intake of milk nutrients would seem to be more important. Thus, some species suckle very frequently (e.g. the pig, at approximately hourly intervals), while others only infrequently (e.g. the rabbit and tree shrew, once daily and once every two days, respectively).

Certain generalizations are, however, now fairly clearly established. Both milk yield (kg/day) and energy output in milk (J/day) are related to body weight raised to the power 0.7 (Fig. 1–4). This exponent of weight is identical to that relating the metabolic rates of different species to their body weights, and since the metabolic rate of the young is a simple proportion of that of the adult, this parallel accords with expectation.

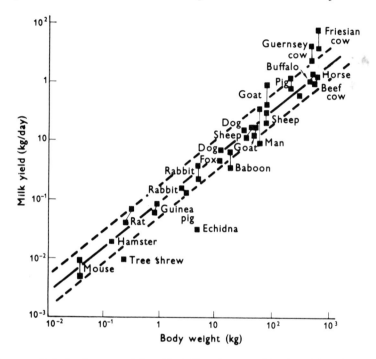

Fig. 1–4   Relation between daily milk yield and maternal body weight. The peak yield has been used, and, where known, the highest recorded figure for an individual of the species or breed. (From LINZELL, J. L. (1972). *Dairy Sci. Abstr.*, **34**.)

Certain species do, however, fall well above (e.g. dairy cows) and below (e.g. primates) the mean line of log body weight versus log milk (or energy) yield. In terms of composition, it has been shown that, in general, smaller species produce less mature young, and that, as would be expected, milk protein concentration is inversely related to adult body weight. Aquatic and arctic species secrete milk with a very high fat content. This could be due to the necessity for the young to rapidly lay down a thick layer of subcutaneous fat as a means of insulation against cold, but it is also likely to be related to the high calorific value of fat when oxidized.

Such examples provide some insight into the factors determining milk yield and composition. The reader will doubtless discern others in the following chapters.

2 Morphology and Development of the Gland

2.1 Mammogenesis

Growth and development of the mammary glands are referred to as mammogenesis. In common with other accessory sexual organs the mammary glands remain undeveloped prior to the onset of the cyclic secretion of ovarian hormones (puberty), but the first signs of their primordia are discernible on the ventral surface of the embryo early in gestation. In eutherians a raised area of ectoderm becomes apparent, running from the axilla to the inguinal region, on each side of the midline. Subsequently cell proliferation to form nodules occurs at specific points along these 'mammary lines', the localization of the nodules being characteristic for each species. Further cell proliferation results in growth into the dermis and increasing protuberance of the superficial cells. The structures, now termed 'mammary buds', grow further into the mesenchyme and develop lumina, the precursors of the ducts and sinuses of the mature gland. At birth the gland is still only rudimentary, consisting, in most species, of a teat and a few short, branching ducts. The connective tissue septa which will ultimately demarcate the gland into lobes and lobules are present, but, in the absence of mammary parenchyma, are filled by adipose tissue cells.

During the period from birth to puberty mammary growth proceeds at a rate equivalent to that of the body surface as a whole, i.e. the growth is 'isometric'. But in certain species a phase of allometric growth, in which the glands increase in size faster than the body surface, begins just prior to the onset of the ovarian cycles (Fig. 2–1). Further development takes place during the recurring cycles following puberty, the extent and nature of the changes reflecting the pattern of hormonal secretion in different species. Where the oestrus cycle is short (e.g. the rat and mouse) growth is limited to extension and branching of the duct system, although much of the development is lost by regression in dioestrus. In species where the luteal phase is longer, e.g. primates, some degree of lobulo-alveolar development may occur in addition to ductal extension, while in others (e.g. the dog and rabbit) the prolonged luteal phase of the ovarian cycle results in a condition of pseudo-pregnancy, in which extensive lobulo-alveolar development occurs and milk is actually secreted.

However, in most species it is only during pregnancy that marked branching of the duct system and lobulo-alveolar development occur, adipose tissue being mobilized to make way for the expanding mammary parenchyma. Cell division accelerates during the early stages of lactation and only diminishes when the peak milk yield has been attained or at weaning (Fig. 2–1).

Assessment of mammary growth is not without its difficulties.

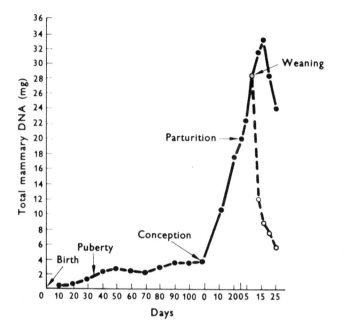

Fig. 2–1   The time-course of mammary development in rats. (From Tucker, H. A. (1969), *J. Dairy Sci.*, **52**, Fig. 1, p. 722. Courtesy of the American Dairy Science Association.)

Currently the most commonly used procedure involves determination of the deoxyribonucleic acid (DNA) content of glands, on the assumption that the DNA content of somatic cells is constant for a given species, i.e. there is only one nucleus per cell. However, it has been claimed that not only is the assumption not strictly justified, but also that it is not possible to distinguish between glandular parenchyma and other tissues, e.g. fat cells. More accurate estimates of the growth of mammary tissue *per se* may be made by combining DNA measurements with determinations of the mammary content of fat and collagen.

2.2   Mammogenic hormones

The close parallel between mammogenesis and the endocrine status of the animal will be apparent from the foregoing section. Indeed, the gland at all stages of its development and activity exhibits an absolute dependence on hormonal stimulation.

In a chapter of this length it is impossible to discuss adequately the work of the scientists who unravelled the complex relationships between the different hormones necessary for mammogenesis, a full account of which would represent a substantial part of the history of classical endocrinology. Prominent in this field was w. r. lyons in the U.S.A., who defined the hormonal factors necessary to transform the diminutive mammary apparatus of the pre-pubertal rat to the fully lactating state. Essentially the techniques employed involved the surgical removal of different endocrine organs (endocrinectomy) followed by the administration of exogenous hormones (hormone replacement therapy) in an attempt to restore the pre-operative degree of mammary development. lyons' results for the Long-Evans strain of rat are summarized in Fig. 2–2. Thus, in ovariectomized, hypophysectomized

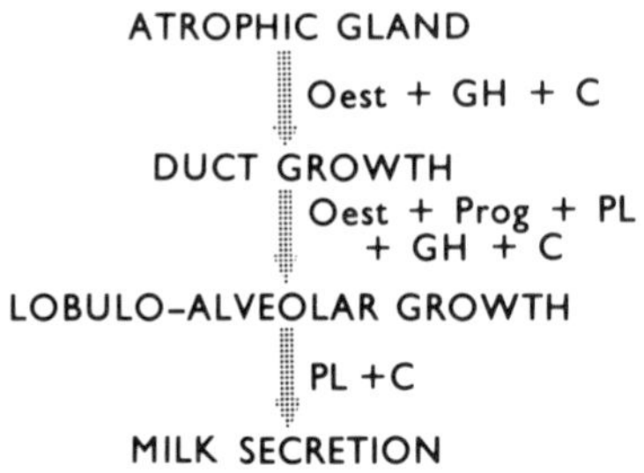

ATROPHIC GLAND

Oest + GH + C

DUCT GROWTH

Oest + Prog + PL
+ GH + C

LOBULO–ALVEOLAR GROWTH

PL +C

MILK SECRETION

Fig. 2–2 The hormonal control of mammary development in rats. Oest=oestrogen; Prog=progesterone; GH=growth hormone; PL=prolactin; C=corticosteroids.

(pituitary gland removed), adrenalectomized rats combinations of prolactin, growth hormone, oestrogen, progesterone and adrenal steroids were capable of eliciting full mammary development. It is likely that during pregnancy hormones secreted by the placenta are also important in mammogenesis. The hormone complexes required at each stage act synergistically, i.e. the development following the administration of the combination of hormones is greater than the sum of the effects of the individual hormones.

While the situation appears to be similar in mice, very few other species have been examined in detail. In rabbits ovarian steroids are apparently capable of inducing some lobulo-alveolar growth in hypophysectomized animals, while in goats pituitary hormones alone may elicit milk secretion in ovariectomized animals. Lactogenesis, the initiation of milk secretion, is discussed in greater detail in Chapter 5.

2.3 Morphology of the functional gland

The basic structure of the mature gland and the division of the mammary parenchyma into lobulo-alveolar (secretory) and ductal elements has been discussed briefly in section 1.2.1. Each alveolus (Fig. 2–3) is composed of a single layer of secretory cells surrounding a central cavity, the lumen. Milk is secreted into the lumina across the luminal, or

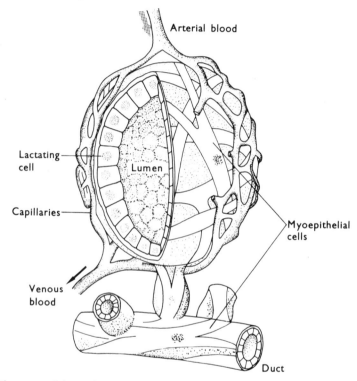

Fig. 2–3   Schematic representation of a mammary alveolus. (Modified from PATTON, S.(1969). Milk. *Scientific American*, **221**, p. 67, Fig. c. Copyright © 1969 by Scientific American Inc. All Rights Reserved.)

'apical', membrane, while the substrates required for milk synthesis enter the cells across their basal membranes. Surrounding each alveolus and lying adjacent to the bases of the secretory cells are a number of spindle-shaped 'myoepithelial cells'. These cells, which also surround the smaller ducts of the gland, branch and form a criss-cross arrangement around the alveoli, so that they have often been referred to as 'basket cells'. The cells are capable of contraction and are important in the 'milk ejection' reflex (Chapter 6).

Substrates and hormones are supplied to the alveoli via a capillary network which lies outside the myoepithelial cell layer and is separated from it by a thin basement membrane. Since the glands are skin structures, the number and disposition of which varies between species, the blood supply to an individual gland is determined by its location. For example, the mammary arteries in cows and goats are branches of the external pudic artery, while in species possessing thoracic glands (pigs and mice) blood is supplied by thoracic and intercostal arteries. The same consideration determines the routes by which venous blood and lymph leave the glands.

Ducts leaving a lobule join with others draining milk from neighbouring lobules to form ducts of progressively larger diameter. The largest ducts draining milk from the different lobes of the gland empty, in most species, into sinuses or cisterns in which milk is stored between periods of suckling or milking. In some species the ducts enter common sinuses which communicate with the exterior via a single teat canal (e.g. in the cow), while in others (e.g. humans and rabbits) each large duct draining a single lobule leads into a separate canal within the teat.

As in the case of the vascular supply, the nerve supply is dependent on the location of the glands on the body surface. In general terms, however, mammary glands receive two types of innervation, viz. (i) somatic sensory (afferent) nerves, conveying impulses from tactile receptors in the skin to the central nervous system, and (ii) sympathetic motor (efferent) nerves, which control the degree of contraction of smooth muscles in the teat and in the walls of blood vessels. The sympathetic system exerts control over the amount of blood flowing through the gland by effecting variation in the calibre of the arterioles. An increased frequency of impulses in the nerves causes contraction of the muscles (vasoconstriction) and hence a reduction in the supply of blood to the alveoli, while reduced sympathetic activity has the opposite effect.

The most obvious specialization of the mammary skin in eutherians and marsupials is the teat, and this structure shows several important features at the histological level which are related to its role in providing an efficient route of transfer of milk to the offspring. The teat is highly vascularized, the veins showing atypically thick walls, an adaptation doubtless evolved to ensure a continued blood flow despite the high external pressures exerted by the mouth of the young suckling. The teat contains smooth muscle fibres contraction of which may increase tonus and facilitate retention of the teat in the mouth of the young suckling. The muscle fibres probably do not act as a sphincter, in the true sense of the word. Finally, there is profuse sensory innervation of the teats, the tactile receptors being highly activated by the normal suckling stimulus.

2.4   Ultrastructure of the secretory cell

Since it is in the mammary secretory cell that components of the blood are converted into milk constituents, a full understanding of the mechanisms of milk synthesis and secretion requires a detailed knowledge of the structure of these cells.

The shape of the secretory cells varies with the amount of milk present in the alveolar lumina, but when the latter are not excessively full, and therefore stretched, the cells are roughly cuboidal and approximately 10 μm in diameter in the bovine gland. It has been estimated that there are of the order of 5×10^{12} such cells in the udder of a lactating cow. Qualitatively the secretory cell is comparable in its structure to that of other eukaryotic cells, but the number and extent of development of the different cell structures (organelles) are indicative of a high synthetic and secretory potential. As is the case with the total number of secretory cells, the internal structure of the cells changes markedly with the stage of development of the gland. The following account is concerned solely with the fully-lactating gland (see Fig. 2–4).

With the light microscope it is possible to differentiate the cell into two major parts, viz. (i) the nucleus, situated towards the base of the cell and surrounded by (ii) a relatively homogeneous cytoplasm, itself bounded by a cell membrane. With the electron microscope, however, it is now evident that the cytoplasm consists of a veritable maze of membranes, which bound tubules and vesicles and are continous both with the outer cell membrane, the plasmalemma, and with the membrane surrounding the nucleus. Much of the cytoplasm of the lactating secretory cell consists of parallel rays of membrane-bounded tubules, which are known, collectively, as the 'endoplasmic reticulum' (ER). Most of these membranes have particles ('ribosomes') attached to them, which gives them a corrugated appearance and results in their being designated components of the 'rough endoplasmic reticulum' (RER).

Scattered through the cytoplasm are numerous oval-shaped 'mitochondria'. These organelles are surrounded by a smooth outer membrane, but within this is a second membrane which is elaborately infolded to form shelf-like pockets called 'cristae'. Attached to these membranes are numerous particles which contain enzymes, notably those involved in the tricarboxylic acid cycle, which is involved in the production of ATP (Chapter 3).

In the supra-nuclear region of the cell (i.e. near the apical membrane) are a number of flattened parallel vacuoles, bounded by smooth membranes, which together constitute the Golgi apparatus. Spherical granules of protein are frequently present within the vacuoles. Numerous fat droplets are distributed throughout the cytoplasm, those of larger diameter tending to be present in the apical region of the cell. Lysosomes, dense structures containing vacuoles and droplets, are scattered fairly uniformly in the cytoplasm.

The plasmalemma exhibits features which differ markedly between the different cell surfaces. Thus, the apical membrane possesses micro-villi, which in other tissues appear to serve as an important means of increasing

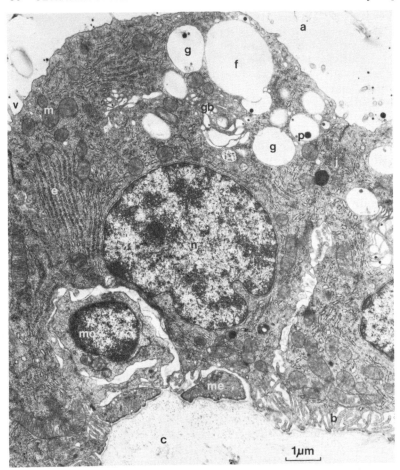

Fig. 2–4 Mammary secretory cell of a goat. a, lumen of alveolus; b, basal folded membrane; c, connective tissue; e, endoplasmic reticulum; f, fat globule; gb, Golgi apparatus; g, Golgi vesicle; j, junctional complex; m, mitochondria; me, myoepithelial cell; mo, small monocyte or lymphocyte (often found in this position); n, nucleus; p, protein granules; v, microvilli. (Reproduced by courtesy of DR. F. B. P. WOODING.)

surface area for trans-membrane transport processes. The basal membrane shows marked infolding to form irregularly-shaped cytoplasmic processes surrounding numerous clefts, while the lateral surfaces are joined firmly together by membrane junctional complexes just below the apical surface. For a fuller account of the properties of cell membranes see Study no. 27, in this series, by A. P. M. LOCKWOOD.

3 The Synthesis of Milk

3.1 Introduction

One of the most remarkable, and ironically, perhaps least-widely appreciated, features of the lactating mammary gland is its high rate of metabolic activity. In several respects this surpasses that of the liver, which is usually regarded as the body's most metabolically active organ. In small mammals the energy value of the milk secreted in a single day may exceed that of the tissues of the whole litter at birth. In dairy animals, in which the processes of natural selection have been amplified by selective breeding for milk yield, the milk secretion rate may be over double that which would be predicted on the basis of the yield of undomesticated species (section 1.9). Thus, a good average Friesian cow with a peak milk yield of 45 kg/day (the world record is 90 kg/day) secretes in excess of 2 kg of lactose and 1.5 kg each of fat and protein per day. Clearly, in full lactation the animal is in large measure subservient to the needs of the mammary glands, which require not only precursors for the synthesis of milk constituents, but also the provision of adequate energy-yielding substrates to drive the necessary synthetic reactions.

It is the purpose of this chapter to consider the substances which the glands absorb from the blood and the manner in which they are converted into the specific constituents of milk. But it will be advantageous to first consider some of the experimental techniques used in studying these factors.

3.2 Measurement of substrate uptake and metabolism by the glands

The traditional biochemical approach to studying substrate uptake and utilization by animal tissues consists of incubating slices of the tissue in physiological saline solutions and comparing the composition of the slices and media at the beginning and end of the incubation. The slices are cut sufficiently thinly to allow adequate rates of diffusion of substrates and respiratory gases into and out of the cells. Where such experiments have employed substrates labelled with radioactive isotopes much useful information has been obtained of the metabolic capabilities of the cells. However, in view of the extensive damage caused to cells by slicing and the artificial nature of the incubation media, it is difficult to know to what extent such data pertain to the physiological situation.

Fortunately, in the case of the mammary gland the relative simplicity of its blood supply, and the ready-accessibility of its secretion, make possible much more satisfactory means of measuring substrate uptake. Several of these techniques have been developed by J. L. LINZELL in Britain.

3.2.1   Arterio-venous concentration (AV) differences

By taking samples of arterial blood and mammary venous blood in conscious lactating animals, and comparing the chemical composition of the samples, it is possible to determine which substances are absorbed by the gland. If determinations are also made of the rate of blood flow through the gland the AV differences can be translated into uptake of a given compound in weight/unit time. For example, if the arterial blood glucose concentration is x mg cm^{-3}, the mammary venous concentration is y mg cm^{-3} and the rate of blood flow R cm^3 min^{-1} then the uptake is given by $R(x-y)$ mg min.$^{-1}$

Several methods have been used for estimating mammary blood flow, of which the most satisfactory is 'continuous thermodilution'. Veins draining the mammary glands of ruminants run along the abdomen close to the body surface, so that they may easily be surgically exteriorized to form permanent 'loops'. Saline is infused at a known rate and temperature (below body temperature) into the vein loop and the temperature of the blood measured with a sensitive thermistor several centimetres downstream of the infusion point. The infused saline lowers the 'downstream' blood temperature to an extent which is inversely proportional to the blood flow rate. Once animals have been prepared with venous loops they may be used repeatedly, over periods of years, for such flow estimates.

Analysis and measurement of the milk secreted during a known period allows calculation of the output by the gland of different milk constituents in mg min.$^{-1}$ It is thus possible to make an assessment of the compounds which are absorbed in sufficient quantities to account for the output of particular milk components. Since only uptake and output are measured, the gland itself representing an example of the proverbial 'black box', the technique, in itself, can only provide circumstantial evidence of the precursors of milk constituents.

3.2.2   Isotope studies

More conclusive evidence is provided by injecting a lactating animal with small doses of radioactive compounds which are suspected of acting as precursors of milk constituents. For example, when glucose, labelled with ^{14}C, is injected into a lactating goat the milk lactose subsequently acquires radioactivity. Although this result indicates that glucose carbon is used in lactose synthesis it does not, in a whole animal experiment, establish the form in which the activity is absorbed by the gland. It is conceivable, for example, that glucose carbon is first incorporated into a glycoprotein in the liver, and that, following release into the blood, this is absorbed by the mammary glands and there converted into lactose.

Knowledge of the fate of absorbed substrates thus requires that the mammary gland be isolated from the influence of other organs of the body. Tissue slice and similar forms of tissue preparation (e.g. homogenates) provide a means of doing this, but in view of the gross abnormality of these systems the results are likely to be of only qualitative validity.

3.2.3   Perfusion of the isolated gland

In certain species the favourable anatomical disposition of the mammary glands, and the simplicity of their blood supply, make possible the use of a technique in which substrate uptake and metabolism may be studied under conditions where the gland is isolated from the influences of other organs and yet maintained in a relatively normal physiological state. Following the induction of anaesthesia, the glands are removed from a lactating animal, the artery and (usually) veins cannulated and a flow of blood maintained through the gland by the use of a pump. Blood can thus be recirculated through the gland, which can be maintained in a functional state, synthesizing and secreting milk, for several hours. The apparatus employed incorporates devices for oxygenating the blood and replenishing absorbed substrates, and for monitoring various parameters (e.g. blood pressure and flow) throughout the experiment. Frequently an artificial kidney is included in the circuit. Figure 3–1 shows a schematic representation of a circuit used in perfusing guinea-pig mammary glands.

Since only one organ is involved, the interpretation of isotopic data is unequivocal. The system, moreover, facilitates study of the effects of factors such as variation in blood flow rate and substrate concentration, which would be extremely difficult to perform in vivo.

3.3   General considerations of milk biosynthesis

Most of the quantitative data on substrate absorption has been obtained from experiments on goats and cows, since the AV difference and perfusion techniques are most easily applied in large animals. Corresponding data for non-ruminants are scanty in comparison, but are sufficient to suggest that there are certain differences in the metabolism of ruminant and non-ruminant mammary tissue.

In general terms, the specific constituents of milk are synthesized from small molecules absorbed from the blood. Virtually nothing is known about the mechanisms by which these precursors cross the basal membranes of the secretory cells. Most of the molecules involved have low lipid solubility, so that, in view of the high lipid content of cell membranes they are unlikely to enter the cells by simple diffusion. Studies on other tissues show that specialized 'carrier' systems exist for substrate transport, in which a protein at the outer membrane surface combines with the substrate, thus rendering it soluble, then moves across the membrane, releasing the substrate at the inner surface. In reality the situation is likely to be much more complex, e.g. there is

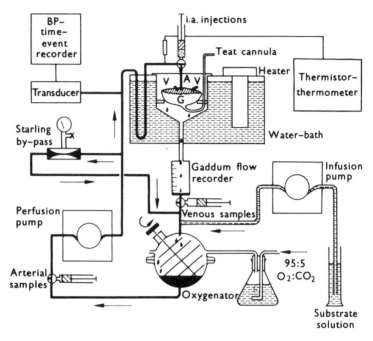

Fig. 3–1 Schematic representation of apparatus used in perfusion of the isolated guinea-pig mammary gland. G=mammary gland; A=arterial cannula; V=cut vein. From DAVIS, S. R. and MEPHAM, T. B. (1972). *J. Physiol.*, **222.**)

probably competition between different substrates for a single binding site on the protein carrier molecule. It has also been suggested that the deep infolding of the basal membrane (section 2.3) represents a mechanism by which extracellular fluid may be transported into the cell following vesicle formation.

3.4 Synthesis of milk protein

AV difference studies have shown that the total free amino acid nitrogen uptake by the glands is adequate to account for the output of milk protein nitrogen, but many individual amino acids do not show a corresponding balance, some being absorbed by the glands in excess of their specific requirement in milk protein, while others are absorbed in inadequate amounts. Isotope experiments show that the former amino acids are metabolized, and the latter synthesized, within the mammary tissue. Protein synthesis involves the assembly of the amino acids, absorbed or synthesized, in a specific order along a chain, in which each amino acid is linked to its neighbour by a peptide (CO–NH) bond. The biochemical mechanisms determining the order of amino acids in the chains of milk protein molecules are apparently similar to those operating in other tissues. Full accounts of these processes, which have been the subject of intense investigation over the last twenty years, will be found in many biological textbooks and a very brief summary only will be given here (see Fig. 3–2).

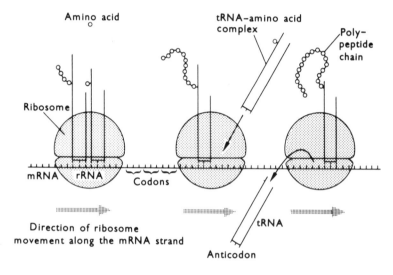

Fig. 3–2 Schematic representation of milk protein synthesis. (Modified, from *Life on Earth* edited by WILSON, E. O. and EISNER, T. (1973). Sinauer Associates Inc., Stamford, Connecticut.)

The 'instructions' determining the order of assembly of amino acids in the protein chains are contained in the DNA (deoxyribonucleic acid) molecules within the nucleus. The genetic material, comprised of DNA molecules, of every cell of the body, contains information for the assembly of every protein which the body is capable of synthesizing. Only part of this information is required by the secretory cells, i.e. that relating to the synthesis of the specific milk proteins and the enzymes required by the cells. The requisite information is transferred to RNA (ribonucleic acid) molecules in a process termed 'transcription'. Three types of RNA molecule are formed, viz. mRNA, tRNA and rRNA. These molecules leave the nucleus and pass to the cytoplasm where each has a specific role to play in translating the encoded information it contains into the production of the actual protein molecules.

Milk protein synthesis takes place on the ribosomes of the RER, which contain rRNA. There is a specific tRNA for each amino acid, the two molecules combining to form a complex. The molecules of mRNA are in the form of long (at least 150 nm) strands composed of nucleotides. Groups of three nucleotides form a 'codon' which is recognized by the appropriate 'anticodon' on a tRNA-amino acid complex. However, it is only when mRNA is associated with the rRNA in the ribosomes that binding of the codon to the anticodon occurs. Each ribosome has binding sites for only two tRNA molecules at a time, so that for the message on the mRNA to be 'read' the ribosome must move with respect to the mRNA (or *vice versa*), in order that the amino acids attached to the tRNA molecules may be brought together in the right order and linked by peptide bonds. The fact that the mRNA is so much longer than the ribosome means that a single mRNA molecule may be read by several ribosomes at once, the multiple structure being known as a 'polysome'. According to this scheme the mRNA molecule appears to act as a computer tape which moves through the ribosomes in one direction while the growing protein chains move out in another, finally being released, in the case of proteins destined for secretion, into the lumina of the ER. Evidence from other tissues suggests that non-secreted proteins, e.g. enzymes, may be synthesized on ribosomes not associated with ER.

3.5 Synthesis of lactose

Isotope studies with perfused mammary glands have indicated that blood glucose is the principal precursor of lactose, though small amounts of radioactivity may be incorporated from labelled glycerol, acetate and amino acids. AV difference measurements *in vivo* confirm that the amount of glucose absorbed by the gland is quantitatively sufficient (indeed, greatly in excess of) the amount required to form lactose.

Lactose synthesis from glucose involves five enzyme-catalysed steps (Fig. 3–3). Enzymes 1–4 are common to several metabolic pathways, e.g. those involved in glycoprotein synthesis, but enzyme 5, 'lactose synthetase', is unique to mammary tissue. As noted above (section 1.7) the enzyme is composed of two dissociable proteins, A and B. The A protein alone, which occurs in a number of tissues, is a galactosyl transferase, catalysing the reaction:

UDP-galactose + N acetyl glucosamine ⟶ UDP + N acetyl lactosamine

In the presence of B protein, which has been shown to be identical to the whey protein, α lactalbumin, the specificity of the enzyme is altered such that the affinity for glucose is increased and reaction 5 proceeds.

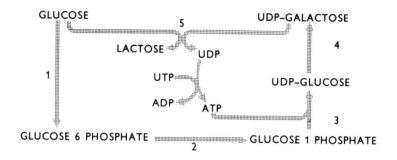

Fig. 3–3   The synthesis of lactose.

3.6   Synthesis of milk fat

There are marked species differences in the chain lengths of the fatty acids of milk triglycerides (section 1.8). Correspondingly there is much variation in the relative importance of their blood precursors between species. Isotope experiments show that in non-ruminants glucose carbon acts as a significant precursor of milk fatty acids, whereas experiments with isolated perfused ruminant glands show only a negligible use of glucose carbon for fatty acid synthesis. By contrast acetate is an important precursor of milk fatty acids in the ruminant but not, in general, in non-ruminants. Micro-organisms in the rumen (the largest chamber of the ruminant stomach) degrade carbohydrates and proteins of food to volatile fatty acids, viz. acetate, propionate and butyrate, so that blood glucose concentrations are much lower than in non-ruminants and those of acetate much higher. Since certain ruminant organs have an absolute requirement for glucose (e.g. the mammary gland itself for lactose synthesis), a mechanism has apparently evolved to prevent its utilization in circumstances where acetate may act as a substitute. The virtual absence from ruminant mammary tissue of the enzyme 'ATP citrate lyase' prevents glucose being used for fatty acid synthesis. In non-ruminants, where glucose is present at much higher blood concentrations, this enzyme is, however, very active.

In all species the starting-point for fatty acid synthesis is apparently acetyl co-enzyme A (acetyl CoA), derived from glucose in non-ruminants and from acetate in ruminants. The principal pathway of synthesis is the 'malonyl CoA' path in which the initial reaction involves carboxylation of acetyl CoA:

$$\text{Acetyl CoA} + CO_2 + ATP \longrightarrow \text{Malonyl CoA} + ADP + Pi$$

The reactions in which malonyl CoA subsequently participates are numerous and complex, involving several different enzymes, but the net effect of the reaction sequence may be summarized as follows:

$$n \text{ Malonyl CoA} + \text{Acetyl CoA} + 2n \text{ NADPH} \longrightarrow$$
$$CH_3.CH_2.(CH_2.CH_2)_{n-1}CH_2.CO.CoA + n \text{ CoA} + 2n \text{ NADP} + n CO_2$$

Following its formation malonyl CoA combines with an 'acyl carrier protein', which is part of a multi-enzyme complex. All intermediates in fatty acid synthesis are apparently bound to this carrier protein. Recently an enzyme has been discovered which releases medium-chain fatty acids from the carrier protein, and it is probable that inter-species variation in the activity of this enzyme is an important factor determining the pattern of fatty acids in milk, which is so characteristic a feature of the milks of different species.

The reactions of the malonyl CoA pathway occur in the cytosol, but there is evidence that other, non-malonyl CoA, pathways exist, the enzymes of which are located in the mitochondria. In addition, β hydroxybutyrate, derived from butyrate in the rumen, may also be incorporated directly into fatty acids in the cytosol. The enzymes of the secretory cell are apparently capable of synthesizing fatty acids of chain lengths up to C_{16}, and, to a very slight extent only, to C_{18}.

Not all the fatty acids of milk triglycerides are, however, synthesized in the mammary gland. AV difference studies in ruminants show that there is a substantial uptake of the triglyceride fatty acids of chylomicrons and certain blood lipoproteins by the gland. The incorporation of these fatty acids into milk triglycerides has been confirmed by isotope experiments, which indicate that they are the major precursors of C_{16} and C_{18} fatty acids. The blood triglycerides are hydrolysed to free fatty acids and glycerol by the enzyme lipoprotein lipase, which is present in the walls of the alveolar blood capillaries. The high activity of the enzyme in non-ruminant glands suggests that blood lipids are also important milk fat precursors in these species. Fatty acids released, and, to some extent, those initially present in the plasma as free (unesterified) fatty acids, are then absorbed by the secretory cells and incorporated, along with the mammary-synthesized fatty acids, into milk triglycerides. In ruminants most of the oleic (C_{18} mono-unsaturated) acid present is derived from absorbed stearic acid as a result of desaturase enzyme activity.

Glycerol required for milk triglycerides is partly derived from the hydrolysed blood lipids, partly by synthesis from glucose, and in small measure from free glycerol of the plasma. Esterification of glycerol with fatty acids is catalysed by enzymes associated with the ER. Glycerol is first phosphorylated to glycerol-3-phosphate and then reacts with the acyl CoA molecules. Esterification is apparently not a random process, i.e. the C_{12}–C_{16} acids are primarily located on the C–2 carbon atom of glycerol, while C_4, C_6 and C_{18} (saturated) are largely on carbon atoms 1 and 3.

Following esterification the molecules aggregate to form the characteristic fat droplets of the secretory cell cytoplasm.

3.7   General metabolism of the secretory cell

It is evident from the foregoing sections that the synthesis of milk proteins, lactose and fat requires energy, which is usually provided in the form of the high energy bond of adenosine triphosphate (ATP). It is thus hardly surprising to find that the aerobic and anaerobic pathways by which ATP is produced (glycolysis and the tricarboxylic acid cycle) are very active in lactating mammary tissue. An account of these pathways will be found in any standard biochemical text. The enzymes catalysing glycolysis are located in the cytosol while those involved in the tricarboxylic acid cycle are confined to the mitochondria (section 2.3.).

Perhaps more noteworthy is the high activity of enzymes in an alternative route of glucose oxidation, the pentose phosphate pathway. In the lactating rat, the glycolytic and pentose phosphate pathways metabolize approximately equal amounts of glucose, but in ruminants the latter pathway is even more important. As in the case of the glycolytic and tricarboxylic acid pathways there is a substantial production of ATP, but a more significant role of the pathway relates to the formation of molecules of NADPH from NADP. Fatty acid synthesis by the 'malonyl CoA' pathway has an absolute requirement for NADPH and it appears that the pentose phosphate pathway is the principal, if not the sole, mechanism supplying this essential co-factor.

Figure 3–4 summarizes the utilization of substrates by the lactating gland.

3.8   Effects of lactation on body metabolism

The magnitude of the metabolic activity of fully-lactating mammary glands is clearly dependent on an adequate supply of appropriate substrates. This supply of substrates is determined by their blood concentrations, the efficacy with which the secretory cells are able to extract them from the blood and the rate of blood flow through the glands. The blood concentrations of substrates are themselves determined by food intake and digestion, biosynthetic processes in the body and the extent of utilization of the substrates by the body as a whole. As a consequence of these interrelationships the repercussions of lactation on the metabolism and behaviour of the whole animal are widespread.

For example, in dairy ruminants the mammary glands absorb two-thirds of all the glucose available to the body tissues, although the glands only account for about 5% of total body weight. The absorptive capacity of the secretory cells is most marked for certain of the essential amino acids; e.g. of the methionine reaching the glands in the arterial blood more than 70% may be absorbed. The supply of substrates to the glands is facilitated by an increased rate of blood flow, i.e. approximately three

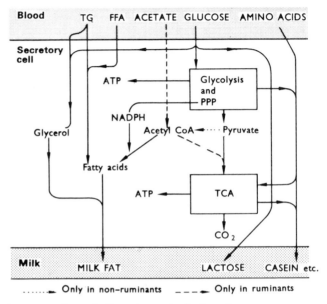

Fig. 3–4   Summary of metabolic pathways in the lactating mammary secretory cell. TCA, tricarboxylic acid cycle; PPP, pentose phosphate pathway; TG, triglycerides; FFA, free fatty acids.

times the rate through an equivalent weight of non-lactating tissue. There is a strong correlation between blood flow and milk yield, approximately 500 cm³ of blood flowing through the glands for every one cm³ of milk secreted in dairy animals. Moreoever tissues involved in increasing substrate supply (e.g. the liver and intestine) also receive larger amounts of blood. Since flow is maintained at approximately non-lactating levels in most other tissues, it follows that cardiac output, i.e. the amount of blood pumped by the heart per minute, is increased in lactation.

All the substrates absorbed by the lactating glands are derived ultimately from ingested food, and it is thus hardly surprising that food intake during lactation is considerably greater than in non-lactating animals. For example, the increase in total food intake in cows may be three to four-fold, while that of individual components, such as protein, may be even greater. Approximately 3–4 litres of water are drunk for each litre of milk secreted. Moreover, in early lactation body tissue reserves are mobilized and used as precursors of milk: most cows lose 5–10% of their body weight after calving.

4 The Mechanisms of Milk Secretion

4.1 Introduction

This chapter is concerned with the processes by which components of milk synthesized within the alveolar cells together with those which simply traverse the cell without undergoing metabolism, pass into the alveolar lumina. We have seen that different cell organelles are involved in the synthesis of the different organic components of milk. The term 'mechanism of milk secretion' thus implies a two stage process of translocation, firstly that by which milk components move from their sites of synthesis through the cytoplasm to the apical cell membrane, and secondly, transfer across the membrane itself.

The most desirable means of studying such a process would doubtless be to make a cinematographic record of a microscopic examination of living tissue. Identification of milk components does, however, require staining techniques, so that one is limited to studying sections of 'fixed' (and therefore, dead) tissues. But if one cannot obtain a moving picture, much information about the secretory process may be obtained from a series of 'stills'. In this respect the technique of autoradiography has proved invaluable. In this technique animals are injected with a known milk component precursor which has been labelled with a radioactive isotope. Samples of mammary tissue are then taken at intervals from the anaesthetized animal, or from several animals killed at different times after the injection, and a series of histological sections prepared. If the sections are subsequently left in proximity to photosensitive films, the irradiation from the isotope will result in the precipitation on the film of silver granules, and the resulting pattern may be compared with the microscopical view of the section, enabling localization of the isotope within the cells at different times after the injection. The high degree of resolution obtainable with electron microscopy (EM) has resulted in its superseding light microscopy for this type of study, and, indeed, for other non-autoradiographic studies of the secretory process.

4.2 The secretion of milk fat

The presence of numerous fat droplets scattered throughout the secretory cell cytoplasm was revealed by early light microscopy. The smallest fat droplets are present in the basal region of the cell, there being a progressive increase in size the more nearly the droplets approach the apical membrane. Autoradiographic studies in the mouse, following injection of labelled fatty acids, have suggested that the esterification process takes place in the RER and that aggregation of lipids to form droplets occurs *in situ*. The increase in size may be due to accretion of newly formed lipid to the migrating droplet surface or to the aggregation of separate droplets.

As the droplet approaches the near vicinity of the apical plasmalemma strong attractive forces (London-Van der Waals forces) are believed to come into play, which result in the droplet being enveloped by the membrane. However, whatever the explanation, the droplet causes bulging of the membrane surface (Figs. 4–1a and 4–2), the close adhesion of the plasmalemma to the droplet surface producing a narrow bridge of cytoplasm between the largely extruded droplet and the cell. At a certain point the bridge of cytoplasm ruptures and the droplet, surrounded by plasmalemma, is released into the alveolar lumen. In the majority of cases the rupture occurs when the cytoplasmic bridge is very narrow and virtually no cytoplasm is lost from the cell. However, a small proportion of fat droplets free in the alveolar lumina appear to have substantial portions of cytoplasm attached to them, often containing cytoplasmic organelles. In the past it has been possible to explain this phenomenon as an artifact due to the juxtaposition of a fat droplet and a portion of a secretory cell in the histological section. However, the association of cytoplasmic fragments and fat droplets in milk removed via the teat (Fig. 4–1b) is clearly not explicable on this basis. It implies that in some cases (1–5% in the goat) the 'pinching off' process occurs before the bridge of cytoplasm between the droplet and the cell has had a chance to narrow. The presence of such 'signets' (droplets with attached crescents of cytoplasm) has been adduced as evidence in favour of the occurrence of apocrine secretion in the mammary gland. Although in higher mammals the proportion of signets is very low, their greater preponderance in wallaby milk (approximately 8% of total droplets) may imply that apocrine secretion in the mammary gland. Although in higher mammals species, and thus provide additional evidence of the homology of mammary and sweat glands (see section 1.3). Many scientists feel, however, that the term 'apocrine secretion' is inappropriate in this context. There can, nevertheless, be little doubt that signets do occur normally in milk, and thus pose a question as to their mechanism of secretion. A possible solution is more appropriately discussed in section 6.3.4.

4.3 The secretion of milk protein

We have seen that milk protein synthesis occurs on the RER (section 3.4). Autoradiographic studies following the injection of labelled amino acids show that, subsequently, the synthesized protein passes to the Golgi apparatus, though the route by which it reaches this organelle has not been defined with certainty. Some have claimed that as the peptide chain is synthesized it passes through the lumina of the endoplasmic reticulum, from which it enters the Golgi vacuoles directly, while others have postulated budding off of protein-containing vesicles from the RER, with subsequent migration to the Golgi apparatus. In the Golgi vacuoles the protein is present as roughly spherical granules (diameter c. 100 nm in the cow), but at higher magnification these granules can be seen to consist of particles 1–2 nm in diameter. Such particles may correspond to actual molecules of casein, the granules being the micellar aggregates into which the molecules form in combination with ionic constituents of milk.

Autoradiographic electron microscopy shows that the vesicles of the Golgi apparatus migrate to the apical membrane, where, following apposition of the vesicular membrane and plasmalemma, the two membranes fuse and release the protein contents by reverse pinocytosis (Figs. 4–1c and 4–2). The modes of transmembrane passage of fat and protein thus appear to be mirror images of each other. This means that plasmalemma lost in the secretion of fat droplets will be replenished, at least in part, by membranes of the Golgi vesicles.

4.4   Lactose secretion

Lactose molecules do not appear to form aggregates in milk and, with a molecular weight of only 342, the molecule is clearly below the resolving power of the electron microscope. Theories on its mode of secretion are consequently based on evidence of a less direct nature than that for fat and protein.

The discovery that the milk protein a-lactalbumin is identical with the B protein sub-unit of the enzyme 'lactose synthetase' has suggested the strong possibility of a close link between the modes of secretion of lactose and milk protein. It has been proposed that while the A protein sub-unit of lactose synthetase is firmly bound to the membrane of the Golgi vesicle, B protein (a-lactalbumin) is synthesized along with other milk proteins on the RER, passes to the Golgi apparatus and is secreted by reverse pinocytosis. While present in the Golgi apparatus it is believed to associate with A protein and thus catalyse the reaction between glucose and UDP galactose to form lactose. Thus lactose would also appear to be secreted by reverse pinocytosis.

4.5   The secretion of sodium and potassium

Mature milk is characterized by a high concentration of potassium and low concentration of sodium. This situation corresponds to that existing within cells and contrasts with that obtaining in extracellular fluid where sodium predominates. Providing, therefore, that the high K^+/Na^+ ratio in milk obtained from the teat also applies to that present in the alveolar

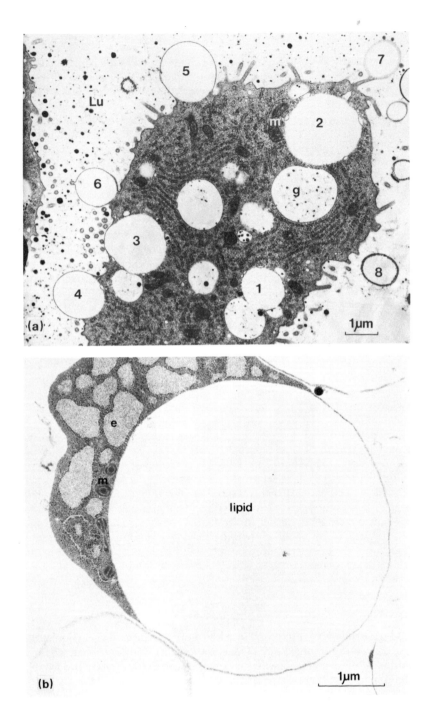

Lu

5

7

m

2

6

g

3

8

4

1

1μm

(b)

e

m

lipid

1μm

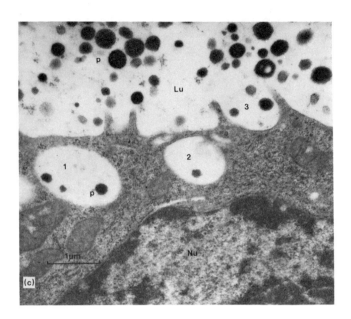

Fig. 4–1 Mechanisms of milk fat and protein secretion. (a) Secretion of fat droplets by secretory cell of goat. 1–8 = suggested sequence of release.(b) Fat droplet from goat's milk, with attached crescent of cytoplasm ('signet') containing mitochondria and swollen ER. (c) Secretion of protein granules by reverse pinocytosis in secretory cell of guinea-pig. 1–3 = suggested sequence of Golgi vesicle migration. Lu = alveolar lumen; e = endoplasmic reticulum; g = Golgi vesicle; m = mitochondrion; Nu = nucleus; p = protein granules. (a) and (b) reproduced by courtesy DR F. B. P. WOODING, (c) by courtesy ANNETTE TOMLINSON.

lumina, it would appear that these ions are likely to be derived from intracellular fluid rather than by leakage of extracellular fluid between the alveolar cells. Moreover EM studies reveal the presence of tight junctions and hemidesmosomes between the neighbouring cells of a single alveolus (section 2.3), a situation which, on evidence from other tissues, greatly impedes the leakage of extracellular fluid.

Living cells invariably exhibit an electrical potential difference (pd) across their boundary membranes, such that the cell interior is several mV negative to the extracellular fluid. The maintenance of this pd is achieved by the operation of 'carrier' systems in the membranes, which transport Na^+ ions outwards and K^+ ions inwards. Since this transport requires energy in the form of ATP, it has been designated the 'sodium pump'. It is possible to measure the magnitude of the potential difference by inserting a very fine-tipped micro-electrode into the interior of a single cell, while a second electrode is located in the extracellular fluid. By combining such pd measurements with analyses of ionic concentrations in mammary intracellular fluid, tissue extracellular fluid and milk, it has been demonstrated that, although a sodium pump appears to be present

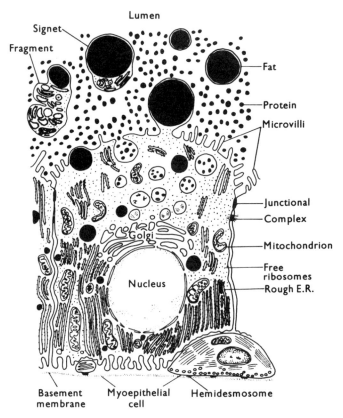

Fig. 4-2 Schematic representation of a mammary secretory cell as interpreted from electron micrographs. (From LINZELL, J. L. and PEAKER, M. (1971). *Physiol. Rev.*, **51**.)

at the basal and lateral surfaces of the cell, it is not present at the apical membrane (Fig. 4-3). This conclusion is suported by histochemical studies, in which the histological distribution of particular enzymes may be defined by staining with chemicals which are specifically reactive with the enzyme under study. An enzyme 'Na+–K+ activated ATPase', which is intimately associated with the sodium pump mechanism, has been shown by this technique to be located at the basal and lateral membranes but absent at the apical surface (Fig. 4-3).

Thus the mechanism which would normally preserve K+ within the cell and extrude Na⁺ does not exist at the alveolar cell/lumen interface and the ions would appear to diffuse across the membrane down their respective concentration gradients. Analyses of the Na^+ and K^+ contents of mammary cells and milk do indeed show an identical K^+/Na^+ ratio in both fluids.

4.6　Secretion of other ions

Analyses of milk and tissue fluid coupled with pd measurements, as described above, indicate that Cl^- ions also diffuse passively down their concentration gradient from intracellular fluid to milk. However, in this case the data suggest the presence of metabolic pumps at both the basal and apical membranes leading to intracellular accumulation of Cl^- ions (Fig. 4–3).

Virtually nothing is known about the secretion of other ions which occur in free solution in milk. Ca^{2+}, Mg^{2+}, and PO_4^{3-} are all present in

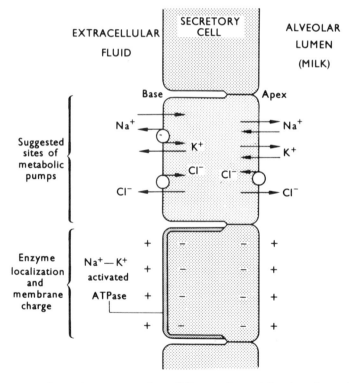

Fig. 4-3　Schematic representation of factors determining ion fluxes from extracellular fluid to milk.

milk in concentrations exceeding those in blood plasma, so that active transport mechanisms for their secretion are almost certain to exist. These ions do, however, bind appreciably to casein, apparently being essential in stabilizing the structure of the micelle, and presumably this binding occurs within the Golgi vesicles. Iron is bound specifically to the minor milk protein, lactoferrin.

4.7 Water

Water constitutes over 80% by weight of the milk of most species. Milk is invariably isotonic with blood plasma, so that it is reasonable to assume that water transport across the apical membrane is governed by the osmotic pressure exerted by the secreted solutes.

Fat and protein are present in milk in large droplets or granules, so that the osmotic pressures they exert will be very small. It may thus be presumed that water transport is largely determined by the secretion of lactose and the free ions. Since lactose is apparently synthesized in the Golgi vesicles it seems probable that water is drawn into these as well as across the apical membrane following lactose secretion. There is, moreover, an inverse relationship between lactose concentration in milk and the molar sum of K^+ and Na^+, as would be predicted if these milk components largely govern water movement.

We have seen that the Golgi membrane becomes continuous with the apical plasmalemma following reverse pinocytosis (section 4.4), a fact which would imply that the Golgi membranes also lack a sodium pump mechanism. It is perhaps useful therefore to consider the interior of the Golgi vesicle as exterior to the cell, and consequently lactose synthesis itself as an extracellular process. Confirmation for this view is provided by the observation that radioactively labelled lactose injected into the gland via the teat canal does not appear in blood, i.e. lactose seems incapable of penetrating the cell membrane in the manner shown by K^+ and Na^+.

4.8 Secretion of colostrum

Colostrum is characterized by the presence of high concentrations of serum proteins and Na^+ and low concentrations of casein, lactose and K^+. In addition, large corpuscles (bodies of Donné), which may attain diameters of $40 \mu m$, are present.

Colostrum results from any condition in which the products of secretion of the alveolar cells are not removed from the gland. Since such a situation results in engorgement of the alveolar cells, it is not unlikely that the tight junctions become broken in some cases, allowing equilibration of ECF with the luminal fluid. This would account for the high Na^+/K^+ ratio and the high serum protein content of colostrum. But serum proteins also occur in mature milk, albeit at much lower concentrations, and since there appears to be selectivity in the passage of such proteins into milk, which is not simply due to differences in molecular weight, it is probable that specific transport processes are operative. At present, however, nothing is known about such transport mechanisms.

The origin of the bodies of Donné has been a subject of controversy ever since their discovery in 1837. The bulk of the evidence suggests that they are macrophages, the function of which is to engulf secreted fat droplets and return them to the circulation, following insinuation between neighbouring alveolar cells.

4.9 Reabsorption of secretory products

In several exocrine glands (e.g. salivary glands) the products of secretion are modified by reabsorptive phenomena in passing through the duct system. It is thus pertinent to enquire whether changes occur in the composition of milk between its secretion into the alveolar lumina and its removal from the gland.

The proposition has indeed been made that milk, as it is initially secreted into the lumina, has a high Na/K ratio, and that during the period in which it is stored in the duct system between milkings, reabsorption of Na and secretion of K and lactose occur. More recent studies (section 4.5) refute this suggestion and offer an explanation of the observations on which it was based (section 6.3.3). Moreover the histological structure of the duct cells (possessing only diminutive microvilli, few mitochondria and sparse ER) differ so markedly from those of organs where reabsorption is known to occur as to be contraindicative of its importance in the mammary gland.

Direct evidence against reabsorption by the teat mucosa of the goat, which is lined with duct epithelium, is provided by experiments in which a light pneumatic cuff was placed around the base of the teat and inflated to a pressure sufficient to isolate the teat cavity from the main duct system, but too low to impede blood circulation. When radioactively labelled Na and Cl were injected into the teat cavity via the teat canal, it was found that no loss of isotope (i.e. reabsorption into the blood) occurred, even after an hour.

5 The Hormonal Control of Milk Secretion

5.1 Introduction

One of the more intriguing aspects of biological systems in general is the nature of the mechanisms controlling their activity. In this respect the mammary gland serves as a particularly useful model because during the adult life of the female its functional activity varies from zero in the non-pregnant, non-lactating animal to very high levels during lactation. Moreover the quantity and composition of the milk secreted is determined, within limits, by the number and nutritional requirements of the young.

The control of lactation is usually considered in relation to two phases, viz. (i) lactogenesis, the initiation of lactation and (ii) galactopoiesis, the maintenance of an established lactation. In lactogenesis some signal of the impending act of parturition must be conveyed to the mammary glands so that the biochemical apparatus involved in synthesizing and secreting milk may rapidly be activated. In galactopoiesis signals generated by the offspring must in some way regulate the activity of the glands to produce milk sufficient to satisfy their combined needs. Control is largely exercised by the nervous and endocrine systems, although mechanisms which are not part of either system also operate. This chapter is confined to discussion of the endocrine control of lactation: for a description of the mammalian endocrine system the reader is referred to Study no. 19 in this series, by EBLING and HIGHNAM.

Most of our knowledge of the endocrinology of lactation has been derived, for practical and economic reasons, from research on small laboratory animals. Since there appear to be differences in the mechanism of lactogenesis between these species and ruminant species, it is convenient to discuss the two classes of animal separately. It is, moreover, important to realize that the term 'lactogenesis' has not been used consistently to describe the same event. The process has essentially two stages, viz. (i) the transformation of the gland from a non-secretory to a secretory state, i.e. in which the cells contain the characteristic milk components, and (ii) the copious flow of milk which follows parturition after an interval of, usually, one or more days. This latter stage is highly dependent on the withdrawal of milk from the gland. The following discussion pertains, unless otherwise stated, to the former phase, which is already in progress prior to parturition.

5.2   Lactogenesis in laboratory animals

5.2.1   Lactogenic hormones

Since lactogenesis normally occurs just prior to parturition it would be reasonable to suppose that there is some necessary connection between the two events. In fact, one of the earliest observations implicating hormonal involvement in lactogenesis was made on animals which were not pregnant. In rabbits ovulation is induced by mating, but even in cases where pregnancy does not ensue, or where ovulation is induced by injection of luteinising hormone, the resulting corpus luteum persists for 16–17 days. The secretion of ovarian steroids over this period leads to extensive mammary development, so that the condition has been termed 'pseudopregnancy'. It was shown in 1928 that injection of anterior pituitary gland extracts into pseudopregnant rabbits caused milk secretion. Subsequently a hormone was isolated from these extracts which, alone, would promote lactogenesis in such animals. The hormone, which was designated 'prolactin', was shown to be capable of acting directly on mammary tissue. Thus, when injected through a teat canal draining one sector of a gland, milk subsequently accumulated only in the injected sector.

The fact that lactogenesis was first experimentally induced in rabbits was, perhaps, not entirely fortuitous. The rabbit appears unique in requiring only one hormone to induce lactogenesis in animals with suitably developed glands. Studies employing the techniques of endocrinectomy and hormone replacement therapy (section 2.2) indicate that for all other species studied a combination of two or three hormones is required. These constitute a 'lactogenic complex' in which the hormones act synergistically. Typically, the complex consists of prolactin, and/or growth hormone, which are secreted by the anterior pituitary, and corticosteroids, secreted by the adrenal gland. As in mammogenesis, during pregnancy hormones secreted by the placenta probably augment the pituitary lactogenic activity.

The principal difference between the mammogenic and lactogenic complexes (see Fig. 2–2) would thus appear to be the absence of ovarian steroids in the latter. This has led to the view that oestrogen and/or progesterone inhibit lactogenesis during pregnancy and that it occurs only following the removal of this inhibition just prior to parturition. If this is true, and evidence for the view is substantial, the question arises of the mode of interaction of the ovarian steroids and the lactogenic hormones, i.e. is the secretion of lactogenic hormones suppressed during pregnancy, or are they, though secreted, prevented from exerting their effects on mammary tissue? There is reason to believe that both mechanisms operate. Largely due to the work of s. j. FOLLEY and A. T. COWIE in Britain and of j. MEITES in the U.S.A., the theory arose that during pregnancy a high progesterone/oestrogen blood concentration ratio inhibits both prolactin secretion and its effect on the mammary cells, while the fall in the concentrations of the ovarian steroids, and particularly of progesterone, at parturition allows the occurrence of lactogenesis. Low blood concentrations of oestrogen do, in fact, appear to stimulate lactation (Fig. 5–1). It has also been shown that, in certain species, injection of adrenal steroids initiates lactation in pregnant animals. The finding that throughout pregnancy corticosteroids are present in blood in an inactive form, i.e. bound to plasma proteins, and that just prior to parturition the binding capacity of the proteins is reduced, causing an increased concentration of the active steroids (Fig. 5–1), suggests an alternative mechanism by which the lactogenic complex may be augmented. Recent assays of hormone concentrations in blood confirm these suggestions, showing that prolactin and adrenal corticosteroid levels are low during pregnancy and rise abruptly just prior to parturition. Furthermore, and equally significantly, progesterone concentrations, which are maintained at high levels throughout pregnancy, fall dramatically before parturition.

5.2.2   Changes in secretory cell ultrastructure

An explanation of the events of lactogenesis requires definition of the changes which take place in the secretory cells of the parturient mammary gland. Electron microscopy of mouse mammary tissue shows that at mid-pregnancy (approx. 10 days *pre-partum*) the secretory cells possess only a diminutive ER and Golgi apparatus, although the mitochondria have attained about two-thirds of the development exhibited by lactating cells. During the period up to and immediately following parturition marked changes occur in these undifferentiated cells. Rapid growth of the ER and Golgi apparatus occur, and concurrently the proportion of ribosomes aggregating in polysomes is greatly increased, a necessary prerequisite of milk protein synthesis.

We have seen that in rats the proliferation of the lobulo-alveolar system begun early in pregnancy continues, and is indeed accelerated, at parturition (Fig. 2–1). Such estimates of growth were based on DNA measurements. Since lactating tissue exhibits high enzyme activity and milk protein synthesis, it would be expected that RNA would also increase in lactating tissue. The ratio RNA/DNA serves as an index of protein synthesis potential per cell and has been shown to increase markedly at lactogenesis. Measurement of the maximal activities (V_{max}), in *in vitro* assays, of over thirty enzymes in mammary tissue taken from rats and guinea-pigs shows that the increased activities of all the enzymes roughly parallels the rate of increase of DNA. The enzyme activities continue to increase markedly *post-partum*, and are presumably associated with the onset of copious milk secretion.

Lactogenesis thus results from rapid and extensive changes which

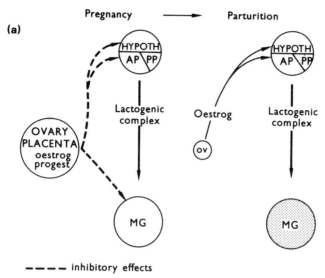

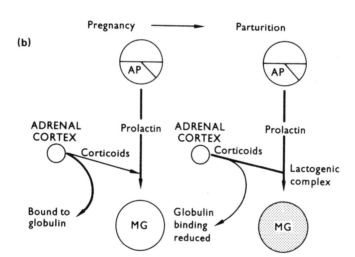

Fig. 5–1   Mechanisms of lactogenesis. (a) Inhibition during pregnancy of the secretory activity of the mammary cells and of the anterior pituitary by oestrogen and progesterone of ovarian and/or placental origin. (b) Completion of the lactogenic complex by an increase in the levels of biologically active corticosteroids. (Hypoth = hypothalamus; AP = anterior pituitary; PP = posterior pituitary; oestrog = oestrogen; progest = progesterone; ov = ovary; MG = mammary gland.) (From COWIE, A. T. (1969) in *Lactogenesis* edited by REYNOLDS, M. and FOLLEY, S. J. University of Pennsylvania Press, Philadelphia.)

occur in the secretory cells at about the time of parturition, changes which are apparently consequent on the activity of a combination of hormones. The questions thus arise of the way in which the lactogenic hormones become effective, and the nature of the 'trigger' which initiates the whole complex series of events constituting lactogenesis.

5.2.3   Organ culture

The technique which has proved most valuable in delineating the roles of the lactogenic hormones is that of organ culture. This involves the maintenance of pieces of mammary tissue (explants) *in vitro* on the surface of a nutrient medium and under aseptic conditions, for periods of 1–2 weeks. The technique requires only very simple apparatus, but considerable care and not a little skill.

Explants of mammary tissue from mid-pregnant mice have been used extensively. As noted above the secretory cells at this stage are undifferentiated, with cytoplasm which possesses few and only poorly developed organelles. However, when explants were cultured in the presence of insulin and cortisol for 96 hours cell division (and therefore DNA synthesis) occurred, and the daughter cells became differentiated. Incubation with insulin alone caused cell division, but the daughter cells remained undifferentiated. Cortisol thus appears necessary for inducing the development of the membrane-bound structures and the distribution of the organelles which is characteristic of the active secretory cell (i.e. with basal ER and nucleus and an apical Golgi apparatus). Subsequent incubation of the differentiated cells with insulin, cortisol and prolactin led to the secretion of caseins by the cells. Moreover, electrophoretic analysis showed that the different casein fractions were present in the same relative proportions as they are in mouse milk.

These results, which are summarized in Fig. 5–2, confirmed the importance of prolactin and corticosteroids in lactogenesis and indicated the necessity for cell division before differentiation could occur. But as with all *in vitro* techniques, in which the cellular environment is quite unphysiological, it is necessary to resist the inclination to extrapolate too readily to the *in vivo* situation.

5.2.4   The action of lactogenic hormones

The action of prolactin in stimulating casein synthesis is inhibited by the inclusion in the incubation medium of Actinomycin D. This substance prevents DNA-dependent RNA synthesis, so it would appear that prolactin acts at the level of transcription, inducing the production of mRNA molecules which initiate the synthesis of milk proteins on the RER. Prolactin would thus seem to be responsible both for the increased RNA/DNA ratio at parturition and for the appearance of milk proteins.

In lactating rats hypophysectomy has been shown to reduce the activities of certain mammary enzymes, e.g. 'fatty acid synthetase' and

'ATP citrate lyase', which are involved in milk fat synthesis, but by contrast to have little or no effect on others, e.g. 'phosphofructokinase', which is involved in glycolysis. Administration of lactogenic hormones to

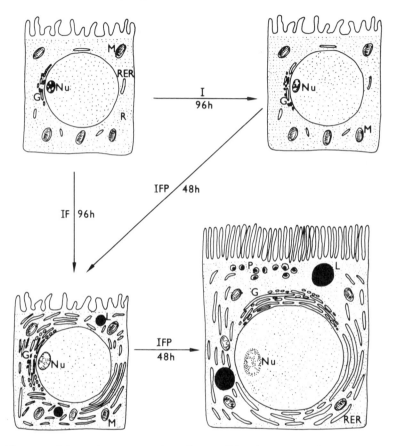

Fig. 5–2   Schematic representation of some of the ultrastructural changes within the secretory cells of mid-pregnant mouse mammary explants, when cultured *in vitro* with added hormones. I, insulin; F, cortisol; P, prolactin. (From MILLS, E. S. and TOPPER, Y. J. (1970). *J. Cell. Biol.*, **44**.)

the hypophysectomized animals partially restored the activity of those enzymes which were affected, and the combination of prolactin and cortisol was more effective than either hormone administered alone. On the other hand experiments with mammary explants from pseudopregnant rabbits showed that prolactin, in the absence of corticosteroids stimulated fatty acid synthesis, the resulting pattern of chain lengths closely resembling that present in rabbit milk. The lactogenic hormones thus also seem to be involved in stimulating the synthesis of the specific enzyme complement necessary for elaborating milk constituents.

5.2.5 Effects of hormones on lactose synthetase

The rate-limiting step in the sequence of reactions culminating in lactose synthesis is that catalysed by the enzyme 'lactose synthetase'. Studies with pregnant mouse mammary explants show that, as for the caseins, induction of the synthesis of this enzyme requires the presence of insulin, prolactin and cortisol. As discussed earlier (section 3.5) the enzyme is composed of two dissociable proteins and the concentrations of both proteins respond to hormone treatment. However, when in addition to the lactogenic hormones progesterone was also added to the incubation media the synthesis of α lactalbumin (the B protein) was inhibited, but that of the A protein unaffected. Furthermore progesterone had no effect on the induction of casein synthesis in the explants. Moreover, assays of the A and B proteins in mammary tissue taken from mice during pregnancy and lactation showed that the increase in concentration of the A and B proteins was asynchronous (Fig. 5–3). It

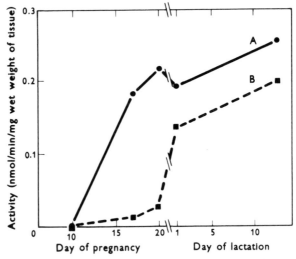

Fig. 5–3 The levels of lactose synthetase A and B proteins in homogenates of mammary tissue from mice at different stages of pregnancy and lactation. (From TURKINGTON, R. W., BREW, K., VANAMAN, T. C. and HILL, R.L. (1968). *J. biol. Chem.*, **243**.)

has thus been suggested that the reason for the delay in the increase in B protein activity is the high levels of progesterone which are present in blood until just before parturition.

Of all the many biochemical events occurring in the parturient gland the secretion of lactose is probably the most significant in terms of the initiation of milk secretion. Lactose is the major osmotic component of milk (section 1.5) so that in the absence of its secretion into the alveolar lumen there would be no reason for water movement and hence no solute medium for the transport of other milk components. The inhibitory action of progesterone on lactose synthesis is thus able to hold lactogenesis in abeyance.

Studies on pregnant rats confirm the regulatory role of progesterone. Ovariectomy results in the appearance of lactose in the mammary gland, which, 30 hours later, reaches levels equivalent to those found at the time of parturition. Administration of progesterone prevents the appearance of lactose in such animals. If lactose synthesis is taken as an index of lactogenesis, the natural lactogenic 'trigger' would seem to precede it by 30 hours. Progesterone is normally synthesized in corpora lutea of the ovaries from pregnenolone, but it has been found that in pregnant rats an abrupt change occurs in the metabolism of pregnenolone, such that instead of giving rise to progesterone another steroid is produced, which inhibits neither lactogenesis nor parturition. Significantly, this change occurs approximately 30 hours *pre-partum*. The reason for the shift in luteal metabolism is unknown, but it is possibly due to the effects of reduced secretion of a placental factor. It thus appears, that, at least in the rat, it is the fall in blood plasma progesterone concentration which constitutes the lactogenic trigger.

5.3   Lactogenesis in ruminants

The mechanism of lactogenesis in ruminants would appear to be rather different from that described above. Lactogenesis occurs in response to injection of prolactin and corticosteroids in pregnant cows and sheep, but unlike the situation in laboratory animals milk secretion can occur long before parturition under physiological conditions. Indeed, it is sometimes necessary to milk cows *pre-partum* to relieve udder distension.

There are virtually no data from culture experiments equivalent to those described for rodents, but enzyme assays on mammary tissue taken from cows between 14 days *pre-partum* and 40 days *post-partum* failed to show any significant changes in the V_{max} of 18 enzymes, nor were there any changes in the mammary cell concentrations of 15 metabolites. Thus, the full enzyme complement is present well before parturition and the sharp increase in milk secretion which occurs *post-partum* in cows would appear to be due to factors other than those operative in rats and guinea-pigs (section 5.2.2.). It is, however, important to realize that the V_{max} of an enzyme is determined *in vitro* under optimal conditions of cofactor and substrate supply. *In vivo*, the capacity of an enzyme to express its full activity may be limited, e.g. by a suboptimal distribution of substrates between the different cell compartments.

5.4   Maintenance of established lactation

The precise shape of the lactation curve (the graph of milk yield against time) varies with species, but, in general terms, the yield rises to a peak in a relatively short time and then declines gradually over a longer period. For example, in rabbits peak yield occurs at about 3 weeks *post-partum* and falls to very low levels at about 7 weeks, when the litter is weaned. The continued secretion of milk is dependent on continued milking or suckling, and is regulated, by mechanisms to be discussed in Chapter 6, to the frequency and intensity of these activities. Nevertheless, even where, as in dairy animals, the milking intensity is maintained at a constant level over long periods of time the yield still declines following the attainment of peak yield.

5.4.1   Experiments involving endocrine gland removal

Attempts to identify the hormones involved in galactopoiesis have employed the classical techniques of endocrinectomy and hormone replacement therapy. In lactating goats hypophysectomy results in a complete cessation of milk secretion, but in some animals it has been found possible to restore yields completely to the pre-operative levels by administration of a combination of prolactin, growth hormone, adrenal corticosteroids and thyroxin. In the rabbit injections of prolactin alone are able to completely restore milk yield following hypophysectomy, but in other species hormone replacement therapy has proved less successful. There are certain problems in interpreting the results of such experiments, viz. (i) where the yield has fallen to zero the restoration of yield following hormone administration may reflect lactogenic requirements rather than those involved in galactopoiesis; (ii) hypophysectomy and similar procedures produce fairly widespread effects on body metabolism and the results achieved by hormone therapy may in part be due to correction of impaired body metabolism and not specifically related to milk secretion.

5.4.2   The action of galactopoietic hormones

The need for continued secretion of prolactin and corticosteroids is, however, fairly easy to interpret. The molecules of mRNA which specifically code for the milk proteins and the enzymes of the secretory cells have a relatively short functional life, so that continued milk secretion depends on their continued synthesis. This factor is particularly relevant in the case of lactose synthetase, which, as we have seen, is probably limiting for milk secretion. Since the B protein of this enzyme is a normal milk constituent, α lactalbumin, it is continually secreted from the cell, and in the absence of its further synthesis milk secretion would rapidly come to a halt. Thus, what, at first sight, might appear to be a wasteful process (loss of an enzyme into the milk) serves, in fact, as a mechanism of fine control over milk secretion.

In lactating rats prolactin has also been shown to increase cardiac output and mammary blood flow, effects which would not appear to be attributable to action on transcription.

5.4.3   Galactopoietic effects

A different approach to investigating the hormones involved in maintaining lactation derives from injection of exogenous hormones into intact animals. A positive response, i.e. the augmentation of yield, or of the yield of a milk constituent, is here referred to as a 'galactopoietic effect'. It has been reasoned that agents producing galactopoietic effects are those which normally limit milk secretion because of low blood concentrations, and therefore that the effect indicates hormones necessary for galactopoiesis.

Most galactopoietic effects can only be observed in the declining phase of lactation. In rabbits injections of prolactin significantly increase milk yield in late lactation, but in cows prolactin is apparently not galactopoietic. Marked stimulation of yield in cows is, however, achieved by injections of growth hormone and thyroxin, or, instead of the latter, feeding iodinated proteins. Neither procedure has so far proved commercially valuable, in the first case because the hormone preparations are very expensive, and in the latter because the stimulation of yield obtained with thyroxin is generally followed by a depressed yield when the treatment is terminated.

In cows which are concurrently lactating and pregnant there is usually an increased rate of decline in milk yield at the fifth month of gestation. This is probably due to increasing blood concentrations of the ovarian steroids.

5.5   Mammary gland regression

After the attainment of peak milk yield there is a decrease in the number of secretory cells, as indicated by a reduction in mammary gland DNA. The decline in milk yield would not, however, appear to be due solely to reduced numbers of cells because the RNA/DNA ratio, an index of synthetic potential per cell, also decreases. Under natural conditions when the young begin to eat solid food the frequency of suckling is reduced. The immediate consequences of reduced suckling intensity are two-fold, viz. (i) the blood concentrations of hormones released in response to suckling are reduced, and (ii) milk retained within the glands exerts chemical negative feedback effects on further synthesis, i.e. there is 'end-product inhibition'. Subsequently other factors may become important. Thus as milk accumulates within the alveoli the intra-mammary pressure increases, which not only impedes further secretion but may also be instrumental in restricting the passage of blood through the alveolar capillaries.

When the suckling stimulus becomes very low marked changes occur in the secretory cells and in the composition of the milk secreted. The engorgement of the alveolar lumina with milk leads to rupture of the tight junctions which normally exist between neighbouring secretory cells (section 2.3). This results in the partial equilibration of the alveolar milk with extracellular fluid, so that milk which is secreted has higher Na^+ and serum protein and lower K^+ and lactose concentrations than normal. Within the cells lysosomes begin to engulf and digest cellular components (mitochondria, fat droplets, etc.), and this process is aided by macrophages derived from the blood. The terminal secretion resembles colostrum.

If glands are milked continually these degenerative changes may be reduced considerably. There are instances of dairy animals having been milked continually for several years, although milk yields reached very low levels in the latter stages.

6 Neuro-endocrine Control of Lactation

6.1 Introduction

A painting in the National Gallery, London, by the Venetian master, Tintoretto (1518–1594), depicts an event in Greek mythology in which Jupiter has descended from Olympus to pluck the infant Hercules from the breast of the goddess Juno. Milk is shown spurting from Juno's breasts, and according to the myth the droplets of milk crystallized to become the stars of our galaxy, the 'Milky Way' (the astronomical term 'galaxy' is derived from the Greek 'galactos', meaning milk). Quite apart from its artistic merits, the painting illustrates, as was pointed out by the late S. J. FOLLEY, two important physiological phenomena, viz. (i) during suckling milk is subjected to pressure within the gland, such that it sometimes, though not always, spurts from the breast, and (ii) although only one breast is being suckled, milk issues from both.

The demonstration of a forcible expulsion of milk indicates that suckling or milking cause an increase in intra-mammary pressure, an effect which can readily be measured by inserting a fine-tipped catheter through a teat canal and connecting it to a manometer. This response constitutes the 'milk ejection reflex', the occurrence of which is vitally important in most species for galactopoiesis. In the interval between successive milkings and sucklings milk continues to be secreted, at a virtually constant rate, into the alveolar lumina, from where it drains into the large ducts and sinuses. Milk in the sinuses is retained within the gland by the resistance afforded by the teat musculature, and if, in an animal with a pendulous udder, such as a cow, cannulae are inserted through the teat canals, much of this milk will flow out under the influence of gravity. Much of the milk secreted will, however, be retained within the gland because surface tension forces prevent its movement through the narrow-bore ducts draining the alveoli. The importance of milk ejection lies in its expelling this 'alveolar milk' from the gland.

6.2 Nature of the milk-ejection reflex

The typical nervous reflex involves detection of a stimulus by specialized receptors, transmission of information on the duration and intensity of the stimulus along an afferent path to a co-ordinating centre in the central nervous system and transmission of information from the centre along an efferent path to effectors, which implement the appropriate response. In a simple reflex, such as the withdrawal of a limb from a painful stimulus, both afferent and efferent paths are purely nervous and the effectors (muscles) are activated within milliseconds of the application of the stimulus. The milk ejection reflex does not, however, conform to this simple pattern. When milking or suckling commence (and this is particularly true, for reasons to be discussed, in animals early in their first lactation) minimal quantities of milk only are obtained in the first 20–30 seconds, at which time the milk begins to flow freely, due to the increased intra-mammary pressure. This surge in milk flow is known as 'let down' by dairymen and as the 'draught' by clinicians. A second feature distinguishing milk ejection from a simple nervous reflex is, as noted above, the diffuse response to a localized stimulus. Milk ejection is, in fact, a neuroendocrine reflex, in which the afferent path is nervous and the efferent path hormonal.

6.3   Components of the milk ejection reflex

6.3.1   The receptors

The teats are profusely innervated, the sensory receptors consisting of bundles of unmyelinated nerve fibres. These fibres are concentrated in the deeper portions of the dermis, in contrast to the rest of the mammary skin, where, although the innervation is very sparse, the superficial dermis and epidermis are innervated. Experiments on rabbits show that mechanical stimulation of the teats gives rise to electrical activity in the afferent nerves to the spinal cord, and the receptors are highly activated by the normal suckling stimulus.

6.3.2   The afferent path

Essentially three types of experimental approach have been adopted in delineating the pathways followed by nervous impulses in the central nervous system. Observations have been made of the effect on the response under study of (i) localized lesioning of nervous tissue, and (ii) electrical stimulation of discrete areas of the brain. In addition, (iii) the electrical changes occurring in localized brain structures have been measured with recording microelectrodes (section 4.5) during operation of the reflex.

Largely as a result of the work of J. S. TINDAL, in Britain, the afferent path of the milk ejection reflex in rabbits and guinea-pigs has been shown to pass bilaterally, in fairly discrete, compact pathways in the lateral funiculi of the spinal cord and through the hind-brain to the mesencephalon, but branch into two, the dorsal and ventral paths, in the diencephalon. These two paths rejoin before entering the posterior hypothalamus, within which most of the electrical activity associated with the milk ejection reflex appears to converge on a group of cells known as the 'paraventricular nucleus' (PVN). The course of the fibres through the central nervous system, and the disposition of the tactile receptors in the teat dermis, strongly suggest that the afferent pathway is part of the 'spinothalamic system', which is characteristically activated by stimuli of an abrupt or alerting nature. This is in sharp distinction to the medial lemniscal sensory mechanism, which responds to delicate tactile stimuli and is capable of accurate spatial discrimination. Thus milk ejection only results from stimuli which, like the act of suckling, are of sufficient intensity and duration.

6.3.3 The efferent path

The pituitary gland, situated at the base of the brain, is in close anatomical and functional association with the hypothalamus. The paraventricular and supraoptic (SON) nuclei of the hypothalamus produce the hormones oxytocin and antidiuretic hormone (ADH), which pass, encapsulated in vesicles, along nerve axons to the posterior pituitary, where they are stored until release into the blood. Release is stimulated by the electrical activity of the hypothalamic nuclei, which is conducted along the same neurones. There is evidence that the PVN is specifically concerned with oxytocin release, though some ADH is also released following PVN activation: analagously the SON is primarily concerned with ADH release, with small amounts of oxytocin also being released. Much of the pioneer work on the involvement of the hypothalamus in milk ejection was carried out by B. A. CROSS in Britain.

Oxytocin injection into lactating animals induces milk ejection at very much lower concentrations than does ADH, and this evidence, together with the fact that the PVN is activated by tactile stimulation of the teat, suggests that it is oxytocin release which constitutes the efferent path of the milk ejection reflex. So sensitive is the response to oxytocin that the most commonly used bioassay procedure for oxytocin consists of measuring the increased intra-mammary pressure following the injection of test solutions into lactating guinea-pigs. The fact that the efferent path of the reflex is hormonal accounts both for the delay observed between application of the stimulus and initiation of ejection, since the rate of blood circulation is very slow by comparison with nerve conduction, and for the fact that ejection occurs in all glands when only one is stimulated.

Recent assays in certain dairy animals have shown that oxytocin is not always detectable in jugular venous blood during suckling or milking, but, whether or not it is detected, milk yield is essentially constant. One possible explanation is that in such animals the capacity of the cisterns is relatively large and the importance of oxytocin in removing alveolar milk thus correspondingly diminished.

6.3.4 The effectors

Although the milk ejecting property of posterior pituitary extracts was discovered as early as 1910, it was only in the 1950s that their target organs in the mammary gland were identified. These are the myoepithelial cells, the 'basket work' arrangement of which around the alveoli renders their contraction a highly efficient mechanism for expelling milk from the alveolar lumina into the large ducts and cisterns (see Figs. 6–1 and 6–2a). In mice the mammary glands are present as flat

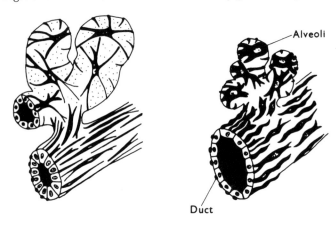

Fig. 6–1   The action of myoepithelial cells in contracting mammary alveoli and dilating the ducts. (Reproduced by courtesy of J. L. LINZELL.)

sheets (i.e. essentially two-dimensional structures) beneath the abdominal skin. If an anaesthetized lactating mouse is placed on a microscope stage and the glands exposed, the contraction process may be readily observed following topical application of oxytocin to the gland surface (Fig. 6–2b). The contraction of the myoepithelial cells produces marked changes in the shape of the secretory cells (Fig. 6–3). In cells in which fat secretion is proceeding concommitant milk ejection may cause premature separation of the fat droplets from the cells, and thus account for the appearance of 'signets' in milk (sections 4.2).

By use of the anaesthetized mouse preparation it is possible to show that the myoepithelial cells also contract in response to mechanical stimuli, e.g. simply stroking the gland surface with a probe. This, so called, 'tap reflex' may constitute an alternative explanation for the apparent non-essentiality of oxytocin release in certain animals: the vigorous butting of the udder exhibited by lambs when suckling is well known.

Under physiological conditions the amounts of oxytocin released in response to suckling remove much of the alveolar milk, but some inevitably remains within the lumina. Injections of exogenous oxytocin at high concentration can promote more forcible myoepithelial cell contraction, but such a procedure also produces deleterious changes in milk composition. In extreme states of contraction the tight junctions normally existing between neighbouring secretory cells in the alveoli become broken and equilibration of milk and extracellular fluid occurs. The milk subsequently secreted has high Na^+ and serum protein and low K^+ and lactose concentrations, and lack of appreciation of this effect has led to erroneous theories of the normal mechanisms of milk secretion (see section 4.9).

6.4   Central control of the reflex

6.4.1   Excitation

When the dam has become accustomed to the act of suckling the reflex can frequently be elicited by non-tactile stimuli. Thus the sight, sound or smell of the offspring, or in the case of dairy animals the environment of the milking parlour, can initiate milk ejection. In such cases the time delay between the beginning of suckling and that of milk ejection is usually not observed. The nervous pathways involved in such 'conditioning' are extremely complex, and no clear picture of the nerve connections between the sense organs and the hypothalamus has so far emerged.

6.4.2   Inhibition

It is a well known fact that in conditions of even moderate stress milk yield is depressed. Since the efferent limb of the milk ejection reflex is hormonal, factors which affect the blood supply to the mammary glands will clearly alter the availability of oxytocin to the myoepithelial cells. In conditions of stress the sympathetic nervous system is activated and the hormone adrenalin released from the adrenal gland. This has a pronounced vasoconstrictor action on mammary blood vessels, so that oxytocin is prevented from reaching the myoepithelial cells in adequate amounts and milk ejection is inhibited. However, in quantitative terms, central inhibition of oxytocin release is probably more important. Such inhibitory processes may well be effective at several different levels of the afferent neural path. For example, perception of pain may block the passage of the impulse at the level of the dorsal roots of the spinal cord, while there is evidence that other inhibitory stimuli are effective at the level of the diencephalon.

Evidence from experiments on rats suggests that even under unstressed conditions oxytocin release may be controlled by the central nervous system. Thus, although pups were observed to suckle continuously, milk ejection, as measured by increased intra-mammary pressure, only occurred at 20–30 minute intervals, suggesting the presence of a central 'gating' mechanism.

Components of the milk ejection reflex are schematically represented in Fig. 6–4.

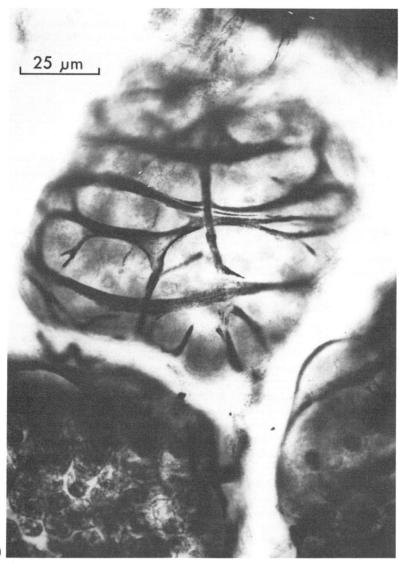

(a)

Fig. 6–2 (a) Myoepithelial cells surrounding an alveolus from a goat mammary gland. (From RICHARDSON, K. C. (1949). *Proc. Roy. Soc. B.*, **136**, 30–45. Courtesy Royal Society.) (b) Action of oxytocin on the mammary gland of an anaesthetized mouse. Left, gland full of milk; right, one minute after topical application of oxytocin to the exposed gland surface (marked with star). Structures running diagonally across figure are a vein (wider vessel) and artery. (Reproduced by courtesy of DR. J. L. LINZELL.)

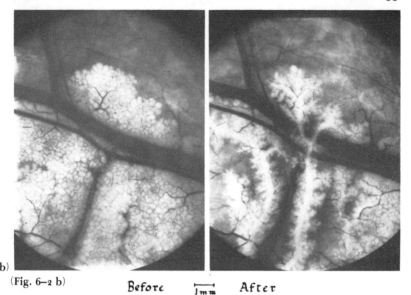

(b)

(Fig. 6–2 b)   Before |⎯| 1 m m   After

6.5   Suckling-induced release of galactopoietic hormones

The importance of oxytocin release is two-fold, viz. (i) it makes available to the offspring most of the milk which would otherwise be retained in the gland, and (ii) by moving milk from the alveolar lumina it prevents the condition of 'end-product inhibition'. Nevertheless, the continued secretion of milk is equally dependent on the provision of those hormones necessary for inducing synthesis of the enzyme complement of the secretory cell. Although there is some species variation in the composition of the galactopoietic complex, prolactin appears to be a universal constituent. Measurements of the blood concentration of prolactin, using a radioimmunoassay technique, show that, as in the case of oxytocin, there is a sharp rise following the initiation of suckling.

6.6.1   The mechanism of prolactin release

Prolactin is one of a number of trophic hormones secreted by the anterior pituitary gland. The anterior pituitary, like the posterior pituitary, is functionally associated with the hypothalamus, but in contrast to oxytocin, prolactin is synthesized by cells in the pituitary gland itself and its release is not directly effected by a neural mechanism. The anterior pituitary is connected to the hypothalamus by a network of blood vessels, the hypophyseal portal vessels, and, in general, release of trophic hormones is promoted by the production in the hypothalamus of releasing factors, which are conveyed to the pituitary cells via the portal

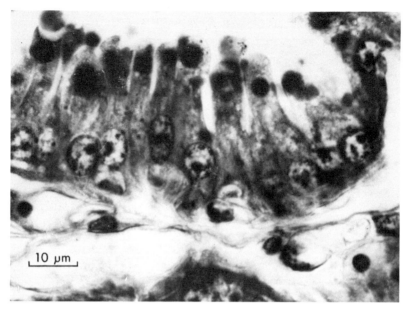

(a)

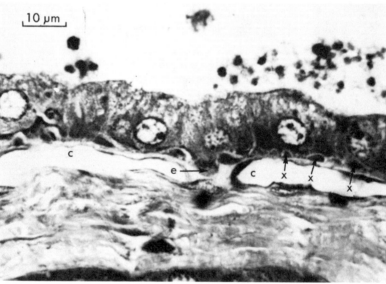

(b)

Fig. 6–3 Conformational changes in mammary secretory cells consequent on milk ejection in the goat. (a) Alveolus full of milk causing secretory cells to become stretched and flattened. c, blood capillary; x, myoepithelial cells. (From RICHARDSON, K. C., 1949. *Proc. R. Soc. B.*, **136**, 30–45. Courtesy Royal Society.) (b) Shortly after milking. (From FOLLEY, S. J. (1952) in Marshall's *Physiology of Reproduction*, 3rd edn. Vol. 2, ch. 20. Edited by PARKES, A. S. (Longmans). Photographs prepared K. C. RICHARDSON.)

system. If the pituitary is transplanted to another site in the body, e.g. under the kidney capsule, where it can readily develop a new blood supply, the secretion of most of the trophic hormone ceases. This is

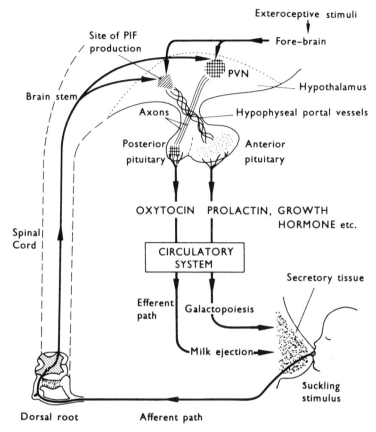

Fig. 6–4   Schematic representation of factors involved in milk ejection and galactopoietic hormone release in humans.

presumably due to the inability of the hypothalamic releasing factors to reach the pituitary cells in adequate amounts. By contrast, the secretion of prolactin continues, and may even be enhanced. Observations of this type led to the postulate that the influence of the hypothalamus on prolactin secretion is inhibitory. Confirmation was provided by experiments in which pituitary glands cultured *in vitro* (see section 5.2.3) continued to secrete prolactin. When, however, hypothalamic extracts were added to the culture media prolactin secretion was depressed. The agent controlling prolactin secretion has thus been designated 'prolactin inhibiting factor' (PIF). Stimuli which inhibit PIF activity promote prolactin release and *vice versa*.

Recently, claims have been made that in addition to producing PIF the hypothalamus is also the source of a releasing factor, PRF. Evidence for the claim is indirect and cannot be said, at present, to be conclusive.

6.5.2   *The neural basis of prolactin release*

Since suckling induces an increased concentration of prolactin in the blood, and a depletion of its secretory granules in the pituitary cells, it would be reasonable to suppose that the afferent pathway involved in its release is similar to that described for oxytocin. Little work has been carried out on this subject, but in the rabbit it would seem that the ascending path from the teat receptors to the mesencephalon is identical to that employed in oxytocin release (see Fig. 6–4). On entering the diencephalon, where the oxytocin-release pathway bifurcates into dorsal and ventral paths, only the dorsal path appears to be involved in prolactin release. The fibres thereafter enter the posterior hypothalamus, ultimately reaching the median eminence, which is the presumed site of PIF production. The exact course of the path from the diencephalon to the hypothalamus is, however, unknown, and it is possible that it passes first through an integrating centre in the fore-brain. There is indeed evidence implicating the involvement of fore-brain structures, viz. the amygdala and hippocampus, which are major components of the limbic system, in prolactin release.

As in the case of oxytocin, prolactin release rapidly becomes conditioned, i.e. elicited by exteroceptive factors, such as the sight and sound of the offspring. For example, lactating rats placed within hearing of similar dams suckling their litters, showed marked depletion of pituitary prolactin, but the effect did not occur when deaf rats were used. Exteroceptive effects may impinge on the afferent path of prolactin release at the level of the amygdala and hippocampus, since experiments in which discrete areas of the cerebral cortex (the part of the brain concerned with perception) were electrically stimulated, elicited lactogenesis in pseudopregnant rabbits. The particular area of the brain stimulated is also known to be closely associated with the limbic structures.

6.5.3   *Release of other galactopoietic hormones*

Adrenocorticotrophic hormone (ACTH), secreted by the anterior pituitary, stimulates the secretion of corticosteroids by the adrenal glands. Assays on several species show that ACTH is released in response to suckling. Evidence has also been obtained for the suckling-induced release of growth hormone, an observation which accords with the role of this hormone in galactopoiesis.

6.6   Possible humoral factors controlling galactopoietic hormone release

In some species, e.g. goats and sheep, release of galactopoietic hormones does not appear to require the suckling stimulus. Thus, even in animals with denervated mammary glands, or in which the spinal cord has been sectioned, lactation can continue, provided that the glands are thoroughly milked. As noted above (section 6.3.3) oxytocin release does not always appear essential in these species. It is possible that, in some, conditioned reflexes based on exteroceptive factors provide sufficient stimulus for galactopoietic hormone release, but other, humoral, mechanisms have also been suggested. The hypothalamus, in addition to its involvement in PIF production and oxytocin release, also contains various 'centres' concerned with the regulation of other functions, e.g. water balance, appetite and temperature control. In view of the high demands made by the mammary glands on available nutrients, it is possible that prolactin release is governed by the action of metabolic factors on hypothalamic cells. It is, indeed, now known that growth-hormone release is stimulated in response to the metabolic needs of the body.

Another possible explanation involves the influence exerted by prolactin in the blood on its own secretion. High blood concentrations depress, and low concentrations stimulate secretion, so that galactopoiesis might, at least in part, be a self-regulating mechanism in these species.

6.7   Diverse roles of galactopoietic hormones

In Chapter 1 theories of the evolution of the mammary gland from skin glands were discussed. It is pertinent, in conclusion, to indicate that those hormones on which the function of the mammary gland depends, e.g. prolactin and oxytocin, are themselves phylogenetically very ancient. Prolactin, for example, has important roles in osmoregulation in fish, in larval development in amphibia, and in stimulating the crop glands of pigeons to secrete 'pigeon milk'. Such examples provide a startling illustration of the way in which, in the course of evolution, the properties of certain chemicals have been exploited to serve apparently quite diverse roles.

Coda

My aim in this short monograph has been to examine the activity of a single organ at several different levels. It will, I hope, have become apparent that attempts to understand the activity of an organ, with even as simple a morphological structure as that of the mammary gland, demand that one pieces together information from, traditionally, rather distinct disciplines, such as biochemistry, neurophysiology, histology and endocrinology. Moreover, the high metabolic activity of the lactating mammary gland, its unsurpassed responsiveness to hormonal influences and ultimate dependence on neural stimuli, would seem to render it a highly appropriate 'model system' in which to demonstrate several biological principles of wider applicability.

The study of milk secretion does, however, have significance beyond its purely experimental and didactic roles. There are two major motivations for research in this area, viz. that of discerning the causes and possible cure of the all too common disease, breast cancer, and secondly, that of increasing the efficiency of milk production in dairy animals. Significant advances have already been made in both areas. There can be no more valid reasons for research than that of alleviating suffering from the twin evils, disease and malnutrition.

In conclusion it seems appropriate to stress the beneficial role of breast-feeding in infant nutrition. In the West the practice has declined rapidly in recent years, but there have been reports recently that in the poorer countries of Africa and South America a similar rejection of breast-feeding is resulting in severe cases of infant malnutrition, due to the inability of many families to afford the high cost of milk-powder substitutes. I can do no better in this context than quote the words of the Roman philosopher, Lucretius, which despite their antiquity (first century B.C.) are endorsed by the most recent biochemical and cardiovascular research:

'Now each female when she has given birth is filled with sweet milk because all that rush of nourishment is turned to her breasts.'

Further reading

COWIE, A. T. and TINDAL, J. S. (1972). *The Physiology of Lactation*. Edward Arnold, London.

FALCONER, I. R. (Editor) (1971). *Lactation*. Butterworth, London.

Background reading

LOCKWOOD, A. P. M. (1971). *The Membranes of Animal Cells*. Studies in Biology No. 27. Edward Arnold, London.

EBLING, J. and HIGHNAM, K. C. (1969). *Chemical Communication*. Studies in Biology No. 19. Edward Arnold, London.

USHERWOOD, P. N. R. (1973). *Nervous systems*. Studies in Biology No. 36. Edward Arnold, London.